HALF THE SUGAR, ALL THE LOVE

a family cookbook

100 Easy, Low-Sugar Recipes for Every Meal of the Day

JENNIFER TYLER LEE and ANISHA I. PATEL, MD, MSPH

WORKMAN PUBLISHING
NEW YORK

Library of Congress Cataloging-in-Publication Data is available.

ISBN 978-1-5235-0423-7

Design by Becky Terhune
Photography by Erin Scott

Workman books are available at special discounts when purchased in bulk
for premiums and sales promotions as well as for fund-raising or educational use.
Special editions or book excerpts can also be created to specification.
For details, contact the Special Sales Director at the address below or
send an email to specialmarkets@workman.com.

Workman Publishing Co., Inc.
225 Varick Street
New York, NY 10014-4381

workman.com

WORKMAN is a registered trademark of Workman Publishing Co., Inc.

Printed in China
First printing November 2019

10 9 8 7 6 5 4 3 2 1

For Catherine, James, and Anthony:
You make my life sweeter.
—JTL

To Iyla, Kasmira, and Sam.
—AIP

CONTENTS

LUNCHES AND SALADS • 69

Lunch Box Favorites

Newtella and Banana Roll Ups

Strawberry and Cream Cheese Sammy

Turkey Panini with Cranberry Sauce

Salmon Yaki Onigiri (Grilled Rice Balls)

Cold Sesame Noodles with Tofu and
   Vegetables

Chinese BBQ Pork Fried Rice

Alphabet Soup

Creamy Tomato Soup

Salads

Fall Harvest Mason Jar Salad with
   Creamy Poppy Seed Dressing

Chinese Chicken Salad with Mandarin
   Vinaigrette

BBQ Chicken Chopped Salad with Creamy
   Ranch Dressing

Strawberry Quinoa Salad with Roasted
   Strawberry Balsamic Vinaigrette

Romaine and Cherry Tomato Salad
   with Miso Dressing

DINNERS • 91

Chicken

Oven-Baked Korean Chicken Wings

BBQ Chicken with Grilled Corn Salad

Chinese Chicken Lettuce Cups

Citrus Chicken Stir-Fry with Green Beans

Vietnamese Chicken Noodle Soup

Stuffed Chicken Parmesan Strips with
   5-Minute Marinara Dipping Sauce

Pork and Beef

BBQ Pulled Pork Sliders with
   Tangy Buttermilk Apple Slaw

Sweet and Sticky Chinese BBQ Pork Roast
   (*Char Siu*)

Beef and Broccoli Teriyaki Bowls

Pineapple Teriyaki Short Ribs

Sloppy Joes

Fish and Seafood

Miso-Glazed Salmon

Poke Bowls

Shrimp Pad Thai

Pineapple Teriyaki Salmon Burgers
   with Sriracha Mayo

Pasta and Pizza

Rainbow Chard Lasagna

BBQ Chicken Pizza

Gram's Meatballs and Spaghetti

Spinach-Ricotta Calzones

DESSERTS • 129

Cookies and Bars

Chewy Chocolate Chip Cookies

Peanut Butter Cookies

Blondies with White Chocolate
and Almonds

Double Chocolate Brownies

Salted Caramel Chocolate
Cheesecake Bars

Salted Nut Butter Crispy Rice Treats

Pecan Pie Bars

Pies and Crisps

Blueberry Pie

Apple Crisp

Caramelized Pumpkin Pie

Cakes and Cupcakes

Chocolate and Peanut Butter Snack Cake

Red Velvet Cupcakes with Cream
Cheese Frosting

Salted Maple-Date Caramel Molten
Chocolate Cakes

Double Chocolate Layer Cake with
Whipped Chocolate Frosting

Puddings and Frozen Treats

Chai-Spiced Rice Pudding

Chocolate Pudding with Maple-Vanilla
Whipped Cream

No-Churn Banana Ice Cream with
Chocolate and Salted Caramel

Strawberry Cream Pops

BEVERAGES • 169

Caramel Coffee Frappé

Kids' Chocolate Frappé

Hot Chocolate Blocks

Pumpkin Spice Hot Chocolate

Horchata

Strawberry-Cantaloupe Agua Fresca

Strawberry-Peach Smoothie

Mango-Pineapple Smoothie

Blueberry-Almond Smoothie

BASICS AND CONDIMENTS • 183

Big Batch Sauces

BBQ Sauce and Spice Mix

Pineapple Teriyaki Glaze

Chinese Hoisin Sauce

Quick-Cook Tomato-Basil Sauce

Slow-Cooker Tomato-Basil Sauce

Condiments and Dressings

Ketchup

Cranberry Sauce

Creamy Ranch Dressing

Mandarin Vinaigrette

Creamy Poppy Seed Dressing

Roasted Strawberry Balsamic Vinaigrette

Toppings and Doughs

Newtella

Nut-Free Newtella

Three-Ingredient Strawberry Jam

Maple-Vanilla Whipped Cream

Salted Maple-Date Caramel Sauce

Overnight Pizza Dough

Pastry Dough

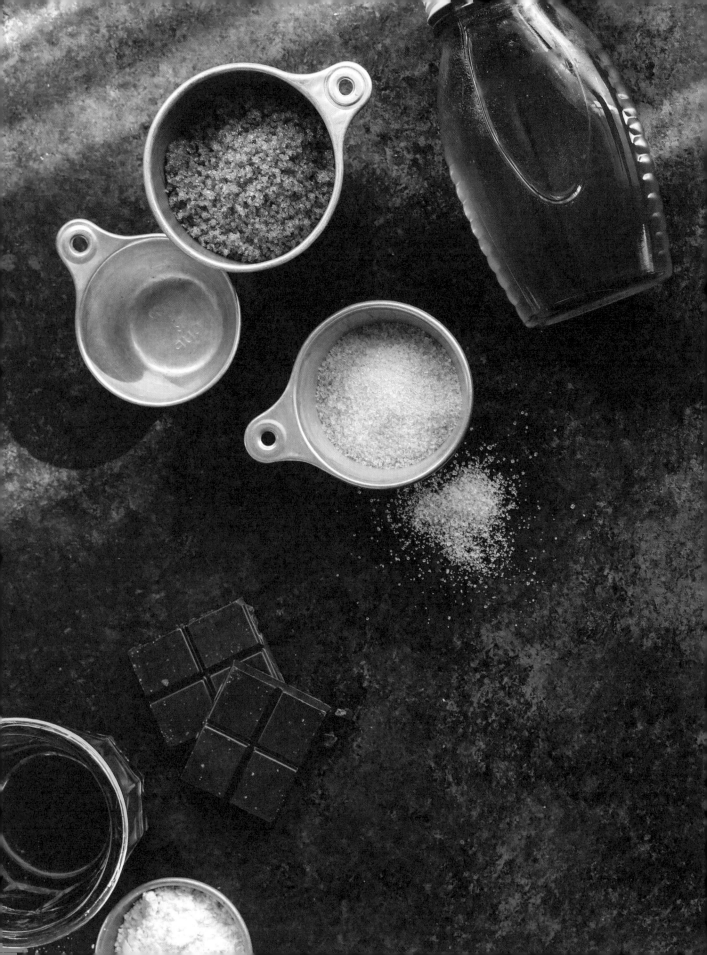

Introduction

WHY REDUCING ADDED SUGAR IS IMPORTANT

Food is at the heart of our families. It brings us around the table to strengthen our relationships, helps our children live healthier lives, and leads to better performance at school. But lurking in our meals is an ingredient that is undermining the health of our families: added sugar.

Kids are consuming their weight in added sugar, about 64 pounds each year. By adulthood, they'll have ingested more than 130,000 sugar cubes—enough to stretch over a mile, more than twice the height of the tallest building in the world. Half of it comes from sugary drinks. The other half is in the foods they eat. Added sugar is *everywhere*, in places we see and places we can't see, and it's putting the health of our children at risk. Scientific studies increasingly point to the health harms of added sugar. It is imperative to change our diets so we can reverse these trends.

Intake of added sugar, particularly from sugar-sweetened beverages (SSBs) like sodas, sports drinks, and fruit-flavored beverages, is associated with cardiovascular disease and the conditions that lead to it including obesity, type 2 diabetes, high blood pressure, and abnormal cholesterol levels. Added sugar can also cause fatty liver disease, which can lead to liver failure. The dramatic rise in these diseases tracks directly with the rise of added sugar consumption. Excess added sugar intake is a major risk factor for preventable diseases that are the leading causes of death in the United States. This trend is particularly problematic among our youngest children, ages two to five years, with obesity rates in this age group increasing at an alarming rate. Consuming too much added sugar is of course also linked to cavities, the leading common chronic health condition among children.

All of us are eating too much added sugar, but children are particularly at risk. Women and children consume more than three times the recommended daily limit of added sugar. And it's not just because they are drinking too many sodas. Added sugar lurks everywhere in our food—in yogurts and bottled salad dressings, in jarred tomato sauce and oatmeal packets, and on and on. Dietary patterns set when kids are young will influence behavior when they are older. That's why it is important to train the palate early to prefer less-sweet foods.

Although consuming too much added sugar can lead to health consequences, people with unhealthy weight and metabolic conditions like high blood pressure, abnormal cholesterol, elevated blood sugar, and fatty liver disease may be able to reverse these conditions by eating a low-sugar diet. Most added sugars are consumed at home, which means that we can take control of our family's health by changing what we eat and how we cook.

But how do we make the change? We can't just cut the sugar and leave kids with bland-tasting food, or worse, add salt and fat to mask what's missing. Instead, we need to give our families their favorite foods—drastically reducing added sugar without sacrificing the flavors they love. The key is to sweeten naturally with fruits and vegetables. That's what this book delivers.

> Women and children consume more than three times the recommended daily limit of added sugar.

ALL ADDED SUGAR
IS SUGAR

CANE JUICE

Palm sugar

Sorghum syrup

EVAPORATED CANE JUICE

COCONUT SUGAR

GOLDEN SUGAR

GOLDEN SYRUP

FRUCTOSE

Confectioners' sugar

Molasses

REFINER'S SYRUP

Cane Sugar

EVAPORATED CANE JUICE

Panela

CAROB SYRUP

Agave nectar

YELLOW SUGAR

Glucose

BARBADOS SUGAR

HONEY

MANNOSE

Sweet Sorghum

FREE-FLOWING BROWN SUGARS

Brown sugar

Maltose

PANOCHA

CANE JUICE

AGAVE SYRUP

HFCS (HIGH-FRUCTOSE CORN SYRUP)

Sucrose

PILONCILLO

CORN SYRUP

CORN SWEETENER

BARLEY MALT

SYRUP CASTOR SUGAR

DEXTRIN

BUTTERED SYRUP

BARLEY MALT SYRUP

MALTOL

Turbinado sugar

DATE SUGAR

RAW SUGAR

Fruit Juice

Dextrose

BEET SUGAR

MALTODEXTRIN

FRUIT JUICE CONCENTRATE

INVERT SUGAR

GRAPE SUGAR

TREACLE

CANE JUICE CRYSTALS

ICING SUGAR

Coconut palm sugar

MALT SYRUP

GLUCOSE SOLIDS

MAPLE SYRUP

DEHYDRATED CANE JUICE

DEMERARA SUGAR

Corn syrup solids

RICE SYRUP

MUSCOVADO

SACCHAROSE

CARAMEL

POWDERED SUGAR

granulated sugar

WHAT IS ADDED SUGAR ANYWAY?

Added sugar is just what it sounds like—sugar that is *added* to foods and beverages during cooking or right before eating. Naturally occurring sugar is present in food in its unadulterated state and is accompanied by nutrients and fiber that help the body process sugar in a healthier way. Natural sugar in fruits, vegetables, and milk is different from added sugar like honey and agave because sources of natural sugar contain nutrients and fiber along with calories. Added sugar is the problem.

For example, if you buy a strawberry yogurt tube at the store, the yogurt contains both added sugar (sucrose from sugar) and naturally occurring sugar (fructose, glucose, and sucrose from strawberries and lactose from yogurt). Similarly, if you make a pitcher of homemade lemonade with honey, water, and lemon juice, the lemonade contains both naturally occurring sugar (fructose, glucose, and sucrose from lemons) and added sugar (primarily fructose and glucose in honey, with traces of other monosaccharides including galactose, sucrose, and maltose). What is most important is to reduce *added sugar*, and that's what this book will help you do.

So where do fruit juices or fruit juice concentrates fit in? While the American Heart Association does not consider fruit juice added sugar, it does classify fruit juice concentrates as such. And the World Health Organization counts both fruit juice and fruit juice concentrate as added sugar. In this book, you will notice that our recipes use whole or pureed fruits or vegetables to sweeten foods naturally with the additional benefits of fiber. This is a healthier way to sweeten. Fruit juices and fruit juice concentrates do not contain much fiber, so we've kept their use to a minimum.

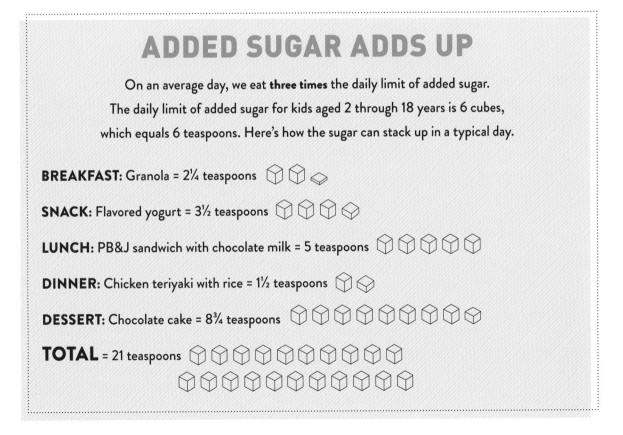

ADDED SUGAR ADDS UP

On an average day, we eat **three times** the daily limit of added sugar.
The daily limit of added sugar for kids aged 2 through 18 years is 6 cubes,
which equals 6 teaspoons. Here's how the sugar can stack up in a typical day.

BREAKFAST: Granola = 2¼ teaspoons

SNACK: Flavored yogurt = 3½ teaspoons

LUNCH: PB&J sandwich with chocolate milk = 5 teaspoons

DINNER: Chicken teriyaki with rice = 1½ teaspoons

DESSERT: Chocolate cake = 8¾ teaspoons

TOTAL = 21 teaspoons

HOW SUGAR BEHAVES IN YOUR BODY

To understand the process, let's take a simplistic look at what happens when you drink a can of soda. Soda primarily contains two types of sugar: fructose and glucose. When you drink the soda, these sugars enter your mouth, where they nourish sugar-loving mouth bacteria. These bacteria produce acid that dissolves tooth enamel, which can lead to tooth decay. When sugar enters your mouth, it also activates sweet receptors that send a signal to the reward system in your brain to take a second sip of that soda. Sugar travels through your stomach to your intestines, where its digestive process begins. An enzyme in your liver processes the sugar and stores it in the organ as fat. As fat in your liver builds up over time, some of it passes into your bloodstream, where it gets deposited in the blood vessels and raises triglyceride and cholesterol levels. In addition, consuming excess calories from added sugar can lead to weight gain, increasing your risk of type 2 diabetes.

FIBER: NATURE'S SUGAR FIGHTER

Fiber helps your body process sugar in a healthier way. Fiber is a plant-based nutrient that your body cannot easily digest. When present in food, this nutrient helps slow down food's absorption so that sugar is released more slowly into your bloodstream. So even though a half cup of fruit punch may contain about the same amount of added sugar as a granola bar, the granola bar, which is full of oats, nuts, and seeds, has more fiber. When you drink that fiber-free fruit punch, you have a large spike in your blood sugar. When you eat the fiber-rich granola bar, however, your body processes the bar more slowly, leading to a gentler release of sugar in your bloodstream that is easier for your body to handle. Fiber can also help you feel full so you end up eating less.

> Fiber helps your body process sugar more slowly.

SUGAR-FREE IS NOT SUSTAINABLE

As evidence on the health effects of added sugar mounts, many people advocate for no-added-sugar diets. But restrictive diets are challenging to follow and are often not sustainable, particularly for children. In a recent study, adults who ate minimally processed foods that were not overly restrictive of carbohydrates, fat, or calories experienced improvements in waist size, body fat, blood sugar, and blood pressure levels. Rather than cutting out *all* sugar or fat in what you eat, the American Academy of Pediatrics recommends a whole diet approach that includes a variety of choices from the five food groups (i.e., vegetables, fruits, grains, dairy, and protein); avoidance of highly processed foods; appropriate portion sizes; and use of minimal amounts of sugar, salt, and fats to flavor foods. In fact, according to the Academy of Nutrition and Dietetics, children on diets do not have healthier weights, have lower self-esteem, and are at risk for eating disorders. It is okay if children consume dessert or even a soda once in a while—just make it *occasional*.

SUGAR MYTHS—BUSTED

There is a great deal of misinformation about sugar. If you feel confused, you're not alone. We've learned from talking with countless families, coupled with our own personal journeys to reduce added sugar, that misconceptions abound.

We are often asked questions like:

How much added sugar is okay?

Should I eat less fruit because it contains sugar?

Is coconut sugar healthier because it's lower on the glycemic index?

Is it better to use sugar substitutes like stevia?

Let's set the record straight and bust the most common sugar myths.

MYTH #1: Honey is healthier.

FACT: There is a misperception that unrefined sugar like honey is healthier than refined sugar like granulated sugar. It's true that a few unrefined sugars have some beneficial properties. Honey, for example, contains vitamins, minerals, proteins, antioxidants, and micronutrients. However, you would need to drink a cup of honey to reap those benefits. It can also promote wound healing and is recommended as a remedy for cough. But as far as the body is concerned, **all added sugar is sugar**. Sugar goes by more than sixty different names (see page 2). Honey, maple syrup, brown sugar, molasses, agave nectar, granulated sugar, and the numerous other varieties are essentially the same once fully processed by the body. Despite the minor nutritional benefits of honey and other unrefined sweeteners, they still count toward your daily added sugar limit (see page 10). The key is to slash your intake of all added sugar—no matter the type.

> Less-refined sweeteners, like agave, count as added sugar just like more-refined sweeteners. In fact, agave is higher in calories than granulated sugar.

TAKEAWAY: Reduce all types of added sugar—both refined and unrefined.

MYTH #2: Fruit has sugar, so avoid it.

FACT: Naturally occurring sugar in fruits and vegetables does not count toward your added sugar limit like granulated sugar, maple syrup, and honey do. In fact, national studies suggest that children are not eating the recommended amount of fruits and vegetables. That's why pediatricians recommend that children eat fruits or veggies with each meal or snack. So rather than cutting fruits, kids should increase consumption! A large orange has 17 grams of sugar, but it comes naturally packaged with about 5 grams of fiber, plus vitamins and minerals. **Fiber is the difference.** When sugar is accompanied with fiber, such as in an orange, digestion and absorption of the naturally occurring sugar is slower so that your body doesn't get a sugar rush. The orange is also packed with vitamin C and beneficial antioxidants. Although many families think that 100 percent fruit juice is healthy, it contains more calories and less fiber than whole fruit. A single 8-ounce glass of orange juice, for example, is the equivalent of eating about three oranges in one sitting with little protective fiber. That's why pediatricians recommend that infants under 1 year of age drink *no* fruit juice and that children limit their daily fruit juice consumption.

TAKEAWAY: Eat more fruits and vegetables. Limit juice.

MYTH #3: *Sugar substitutes are a smarter choice.*

FACT: Artificial sweeteners including aspartame (NutraSweet, Equal), saccharin (Sweet'N Low), and sucralose (Splenda) are often used to cut calories, but there is limited evidence that these sugar substitutes improve health, and their health harms cannot be ignored. Artificial sweeteners tell the "sweet center" in your brain that sugar is coming. But when no sugar or calories follow, it may leave your brain craving more. Consuming artificial sweeteners that taste even sweeter than sugar may also lead to preferences for sweet foods. In addition, artificial sweeteners may upset the balance of healthy bacteria in your gut that can play a role in obesity and other health problems. Stevia, a natural sugar substitute, has not been fully evaluated by the Food and Drug Administration (FDA), and there are no long-term evaluations of the health impacts of its consumption. The FDA has set acceptable daily intake (ADI) levels for more long-standing sugar substitutes, but given the lack of data on the long-term health benefits and harms of these sweeteners, we recommend avoiding them, particularly among children.

TAKEAWAY: Avoid sugar substitutes.

MYTH #4: *No added sugar means no dessert.*

FACT: Dessert isn't the only source of added sugar. Less than a quarter of added sugar intake comes from desserts and candy. Half of added sugar intake comes from beverages. Another 20 percent comes from hidden sugar like that in condiments, dressings, and sauces. Sugar sneaks in everywhere. That's why it's important to reduce added sugar in all of your meals, not just dessert, to reduce how much of it you are consuming. But that doesn't mean you have to give up the foods you love. The secret is learning the hacks for sweetening foods naturally with flavorful whole ingredients like fruits, vegetables, or nuts and seeds. As any experienced cook knows, added sugar plays a key role in flavor and texture. And we don't want to see salt and fat in the place of the added sugar we've cut. This book will arm you with clever strategies to whip up recipes that are delicious and full of flavor, but that also meet a doctor's approval so you can continue to enjoy your favorites in a healthier way.

TAKEAWAY: Use naturally sweet fruits, vegetables, nuts, seeds, and spices to provide flavor with less added sugar.

MYTH #5: *Most families keep added sugar in check.*

FACT: Most parents think that their families are eating healthily, but they're surprised when they learn that women and children are consuming three times the daily recommended limit for added sugar. Those organic fruit gummies, wholesome protein bars, and all-natural prepared foods you buy from your favorite grocery store are often packed with added sugar and hidden behind a "healthy" label. Just a bowl of all-natural granola can put your child over his or her daily added sugar limit at breakfast. Sugar is lurking everywhere. It's in obvious foods like cookies, cakes, and candy, and "concealed" in products like sauces and salad dressings, breads and crackers, breakfast cereals and flavored oatmeal, frozen pizzas, canned soups, condiments, and yogurts. And it adds up, fast.

TAKEAWAY: Learn how to read food labels to spot hidden sugar. See How to Read a Food Label (opposite).

HOW TO READ A FOOD LABEL

With the current nutrition label, it's challenging to know how much added sugar is in packaged foods. Most labels do not show how much of the total sugar in food comes from added sugar. The FDA mandated updated nutrition labels that list the grams of added sugar, but the introduction of these new labels has been delayed. At the time of this writing, those updated nutrition labels are not yet fully in effect. There is a way, though, to estimate added sugar even when it's not listed. Here's how.

Say you eat a 1-cup serving of vanilla yogurt. The package lists 29 grams of total sugar. There are two types of sugar in the yogurt—naturally occurring lactose in the dairy and granulated sugar, or sucrose, that is used to sweeten the yogurt. Here's how to calculate the number of teaspoons of sucrose, which is the *added sugar* in the yogurt:

STEP 1: Compare vanilla yogurt (sweetened with sucrose) to plain yogurt (unsweetened—no sucrose but containing lactose).

29 GRAMS IN VANILLA YOGURT VERSUS 15 GRAMS IN PLAIN YOGURT

STEP 2: Subtract the sugar in the plain yogurt from the sugar in the sweetened yogurt.

29 GRAMS–15 GRAMS = 14 GRAMS ADDED SUGAR (FROM SUCROSE)

STEP 3: Divide grams by 4 to get to teaspoons. (Granulated sugar contains 4.2 grams of sugar per teaspoon, but for ease of calculating you can round to 4 grams. For more on this, see page 11.)

14 GRAMS ÷ 4 = 3½ TEASPOONS ADDED SUGAR PER SERVING

VANILLA YOGURT

Nutrition Facts
Serving Size 1 cup (227g)
Servings Per Container About 4

Amount Per Serving

Calories 170	Calories from Fat 20

	% Daily Value*
Total Fat 2g	**3%**
Saturated Fat 1.5g	**8%**
Trans Fat 0g	
Cholesterol 10mg	**3%**
Sodium 130mg	**5%**
Potassium 440mg	**13%**
Total Carbohydrate 29g	**10%**
Dietary Fiber 0g	**0%**
Sugars 29g	
Protein 9g	**18%**

Vitamin A	2%	•	Vitamin C	0%
Calcium	35%	•	Iron	0%
Vitamin D	25%			

PLAIN YOGURT

Nutrition Facts
Serving Size 1 cup (227g)
Servings Per Container About 4

Amount Per Serving

Calories 120	Calories from Fat 20

	% Daily Value*
Total Fat 2g	**3%**
Saturated Fat 1.5g	**8%**
Trans Fat 0g	
Cholesterol 15mg	**5%**
Sodium 140mg	**6%**
Potassium 480mg	**14%**
Total Carbohydrate 15g	**5%**
Dietary Fiber 0g	**0%**
Sugars 15g	
Protein 10g	**20%**

Vitamin A	2%	•	Vitamin C	0%
Calcium	35%	•	Iron	0%
Vitamin D	25%			

7 SIMPLE TIPS FOR REDUCING ADDED SUGAR

Staying within your daily limit of added sugar is easier if you follow this advice.

1. COOK MORE. The easiest way to reduce added sugar is to cook at home when you can. Most fast foods and processed foods contain added sugar—often when you don't expect it. Cooking helps you regain control over what you eat.

2. SWEETEN NATURALLY. Ripe, in-season fruits and vegetables can sweeten your favorite recipes with less (or no) added sugar. Nectarines can flavor BBQ sauce (page 185), dates can replace sugar in cookies (pages 131 and 133), and caramelized pumpkin or banana can sweeten breads (pages 51 and 52) and pies (page 148). Fruits and vegetables contain fiber that allows for healthier processing of sugar by your body.

3. SPICE IT UP. Spices like cinnamon, cardamom, and vanilla help boost flavor so you can reduce added sugar. Toasted nuts and seeds can add texture and flavor, too.

4. DRINK WATER. Drinking water instead of sugary drinks can dramatically reduce intake of added sugar and calories and can prevent unhealthy weight gain and cavities. It can also help increase hydration to promote learning. Add fruits—like sliced lemons, limes, and oranges—to infuse water with flavor and make it fun (see page 180). Keep a pitcher of chilled water in the fridge. Make sure everyone in your family has their own water bottle (or sippy cup) so they can drink water on the go. Save sugary drinks and juice for special occasions—limit them to once a week.

5. START YOUR DAY RIGHT. Eating a healthy breakfast can promote learning and academic performance. But many breakfast foods, such as cereals, flavored yogurt, and energy bars, can put your family over their daily added sugar limit by midmorning. For breakfast, choose foods that are low in sugar and high in fiber and protein. Plain yogurt with fresh fruit, unsweetened nut butter on whole-wheat toast, and eggs are a few examples. Choose unsweetened milk and fruit instead of flavored milk and juice (even freshly squeezed).

6. SHOP SMART. When purchasing packaged foods, always read the nutrition label (see page 7). Remember, there are about 4 grams in 1 teaspoon of sugar. And don't forget to take into account the serving size, too. Learn to spot the foods where added sugar hides and identify sugar's many aliases (see page 2). Avoid sugar substitutes. Choose unsweetened products when possible. Try not to buy sugar-laden foods. A simple rule: If you want a treat, make it at home.

7. BE FLEXIBLE. If you exceed your daily added sugar limit, it's okay. Just try to reduce added sugar intake during other days of the week to get back in balance and stay below your added sugar targets for the rest of the week.

HOW MUCH FRUIT JUICE IS OKAY?

Less than 1 year of age = no juice unless clinically indicated, like for constipation
1 to 3 years old = 4 ounces/day
4 to 6 years old = 4 to 6 ounces/day
7 to 18 years old = 8 ounces/day
It's best to have fruit and water instead of juice and limit drinks with added sugar to once a week as a special treat.

A GUIDE TO *HALF THE SUGAR, ALL THE LOVE* COOKING

Our recipes make it easy for you to eat what you love with less added sugar and more flavor. We've designed a simple game plan to help you track how much added sugar you're eating each day. Here's how it works.

1. KNOW YOUR TARGET: Based on their age and gender, every member of your family has a recommended maximum amount of added sugar he or she should consume each day (see page 10). This is your daily target.

2. SPOT THE CUBES: Every recipe in this book has sugar cube icons that show the amount of added sugar per serving relative to a leading brand's packaged product or a typical recipe (when a packaged product was not available). Each cube equals 1 teaspoon of sugar. The total number of cubes represents the amount of added sugar in "Theirs"; the pink shaded cubes show the amount in "Ours."

For example, the recipe for Double Chocolate Layer Cake with Whipped Chocolate Frosting (page 158) shows added sugar per serving for "Ours" (3¾ teaspoons) based on the ingredients used in the recipe and compares to "Theirs" (10 to 12 teaspoons), which is the total added sugar per serving in a leading national brand. Recipes with zero added sugar or a negligible amount will also have a ⊗ icon (those with a negligible amount will be indicated as such).

3. COUNT THE CUBES: Recipes can be combined any way you like. Just be mindful of how the cubes are stacking up throughout the day. Most days you'll stay within your limit. There will be occasions, like birthdays and holidays, when you'll indulge—and that's okay! If you go over your added sugar limit for the day, just eat less added sugar for a while to recalibrate.

This recipe = 3¾ teaspoons

DOUBLE CHOCOLATE LAYER CAKE
WITH WHIPPED CHOCOLATE FROSTING

OURS: 3¾ TEASPOONS
THEIRS: 10 TO 12 TEASPOONS

Ingredients

Nonstick cooking spray
1⅓ cups all-purpose flour
½ cup unsweetened natural cocoa powder
1½ teaspoons baking powder
1½ teaspoons salt
1 teaspoon baking soda
½ cup (1 stick) unsalted butter, at room temperature
⅓ cup sugar
2 large eggs
1 tablespoon pure vanilla extract
¾ cup whole milk
1 cup freshly brewed coffee, cooled slightly
2 teaspoons white vinegar
Whipped Chocolate Frosting (recipe follows)
Flaky sea salt, for garnish (optional)

SERVES 12

Rich and ultra chocolaty layers of chocolate cake are paired with whipped chocolate frosting for a decadent treat. Coffee adds a hint of robust flavor while also enhancing the intense chocolate flavor of unsweetened cocoa powder. It's the secret ingredient that pulls it all together. The cake layers are not as thick as those of a typical layer cake, but they are intense! When paired with a fluffy whipped chocolate frosting, this cake is beautifully balanced. It's perfect for your most special celebrations.

1 Preheat the oven to 350°F. Coat two 8-inch round cake pans with cooking spray. Line with parchment paper and coat the parchment paper with cooking spray.

2 Combine the flour, cocoa powder, baking powder, salt, and baking soda in a medium bowl; set aside.

3 Beat the butter and sugar on medium speed in the bowl of of a stand mixer fitted with a paddle attachment until light and fluffy, about 3 minutes. Add the eggs one at a time, beating after each addition. Add the vanilla, increase the speed to medium-high, and beat for 30 seconds.

4 Add the flour mixture in three additions, alternating with the milk, and beat on medium speed until just combined. With the mixer on low speed, slowly pour in the warm coffee. Once it is mostly incorporated, add the vinegar, increase the speed to medium-high, and beat for 30 seconds, scraping the bowl as needed.

5 Divide the batter evenly between the prepared cake pans and bake until a toothpick inserted into the center of each cake comes out clean, about 30 minutes. Let the cakes cool in the pans for 10 minutes, then remove the cakes from the pans and transfer them to a wire rack to cool completely.

Recipe continues

YOUR DAILY TARGET OF ADDED SUGAR

Children younger than 2 years = 0 teaspoons

Children 2 to 18 years = 6 teaspoons

Women (18+) = 6 teaspoons

Men (18+) = 9 teaspoons

ABOUT OUR RECIPES

Our goal is to help you and your family reduce your added sugar consumption by half, if not more. All the recipes in this book contain *at least* 50 percent less added sugar than their comparable recipes, and in some cases much less or no added sugar at all. Since all added sugar is sugar—remember that honey, agave, maple syrup, and other unrefined sweeteners count as added sugar—we use the type of added sugar that achieves the best results for each recipe. Sometimes it's honey and sometimes it's granulated sugar, but it's always kept to a minimum. Our recipes incorporate naturally sweet fruits and vegetables to boost flavor with less or no added sugar, and more vitamins, minerals, and fiber. For example, our Chewy Chocolate Chip Cookies (page 131) are sweetened with naturally sweet dates and no-added-sugar vanilla extract to add flavor without added sugar. They also need a touch of brown sugar to achieve that quintessential chocolate chip cookie flavor, so we use it sparingly. The result: an irresistible chocolate chip cookie with 50 percent less added sugar than a classic chocolate chip cookie.

NUTRITION GUIDELINES

Reducing added sugar while balancing sodium and saturated fat is important for health. You can't slash added sugar and load up on fat and salt to mask the change. We've included our guidelines for keeping these three macronutrients in check. Occasionally you'll enjoy a meal or dessert that falls outside these boundaries, and that's okay! Simply try to adjust your meals throughout the week to compensate.

ADDED SUGAR TARGETS: We rely on daily added sugar guidelines from the American Heart Association, which are most commonly used in the United States: up to 6 teaspoons for children 2 to 18 years old, 6 teaspoons for women, and 9 teaspoons for men. Guidelines also advise that children under the age of 2 years should not consume any foods or beverages with added sugar, including sugar-sweetened drinks.

For our nutrition analysis, we used the following methodology:

First, we calculated added sugar per serving in grams, based on the type of added sugar(s) used in the recipe. Then we converted grams to teaspoons based on grams of sugar per type of added sugar (see Box, opposite page). For example, granulated sugar is 4.2 grams per teaspoon versus honey, which is 5.8 grams per teaspoon.

For product comparisons, when nutrition labels did not list added sugar, we used the following estimate: 4 grams added sugar = 1 teaspoon added sugar.

Added sugar estimates are rounded to the nearest quarter-teaspoon.

Nutrition data used for calculations is primarily from the United States Department of Agriculture (USDA) databases, specifically the National Nutrient Database for Standard Reference and the Food and Nutrient Database for Dietary Studies.

SODIUM TARGETS: The American Heart Association recommends 1,500 mg or less of sodium a day for all Americans for ideal heart health. We use this conservative target as our lower limit for both adults and children. Federal Dietary Guidelines serve as our upper bound.

Note that 1 teaspoon of salt equals 2,300 mg.

1 to 3 years old	1,500 mg
4 to 8 years old	1,500 mg to 1,900 mg
9 to 13 years old	1,500 mg to 2,200 mg
14 to 18 years old	1,500 mg to 2,300 mg
Women (18+)	1,500 mg to 2,300 mg
Men (18+)	1,500 mg to 2,300 mg

SATURATED FAT TARGETS: It's best if most of your fats are healthy fats—polyunsaturated and monounsaturated fatty acids—such as those found in nuts and fish and vegetable oils. Note that we allow exceedances for fat when nuts are used due to their added nutritional benefits. A rough rule is 20 grams or less of saturated fat per day with zero grams of trans fat. For both children and adults, keep saturated fats to 10 percent of total calories per day.

GRAMS OF SUGAR PER TYPE OF ADDED SUGAR

Grams of sugar vary widely by type of added sugar. Honey, for example, has more grams of sugar per teaspoon than granulated sugar. That means you can't swap them 1:1. When calculating teaspoons of added sugar in our recipes, we have accounted for these differences.

TYPE	GRAMS OF SUGAR PER CUP	GRAMS OF SUGAR PER TEASPOON
Granulated sugar	200	4.2
Brown sugar (packed)	213	4.4
Confectioners' sugar (unsifted)	117	2.4
Maple syrup	190	4
Molasses	252	5.3
Light corn syrup	262	5.5
Honey	278	5.8
Semisweet chocolate	93	1.9
Dark chocolate*	62	1.3
White chocolate	99	2.1

* Added sugar varies widely in dark chocolate. We used USDA code 19903 (Chocolate, dark, 60–69% cacao solids) for our nutrition analysis.

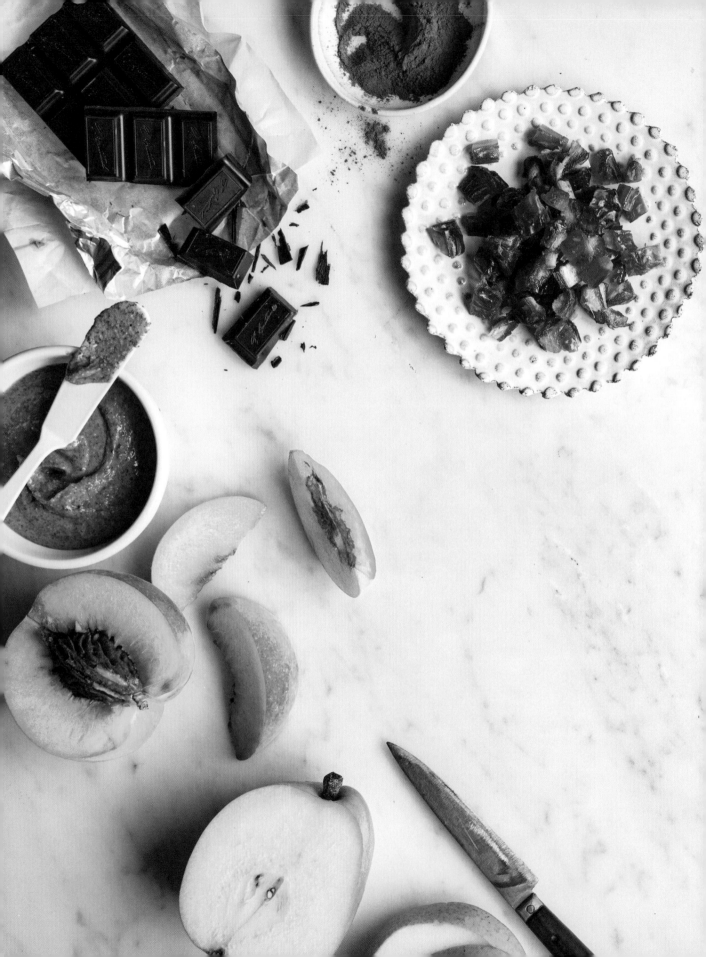

KEY INGREDIENTS

It took a tremendous amount of experimentation to develop delicious recipes with at least 50 percent less added sugar than the original. We learned that there are several key ingredients that are essential to cooking and baking successfully with less added sugar. These ingredients, available in most well-stocked grocery stores, preserve texture and add flavor so you don't miss the sugar one bit.

DATES: These chewy little fruits are essential to low-sugar cooking. They are packed with natural sweetness and caramel-like flavor, and each date contains about 1.6 grams of fiber. Unless otherwise specified, our preference is Medjool dates for their soft texture and sweet flavor. You'll find them in the fresh produce aisle. Use Deglet Noor dates—smaller, firmer, more easily found at your local grocery store, and less expensive—in a pinch.

RIPE FRUITS: Dark speckled bananas, in-season summer berries, sweet apples and pears, and juicy stone fruits are featured throughout our recipes. Be sure to use very ripe fruits to maximize their natural sugars.

CANNED FRUITS AND VEGETABLES: Canned pumpkin, sweet potato, and pineapple are helpful not only because they can be used to sweeten but also because they're handy, shelf-stable shortcuts.

SPICES: Vanilla, cinnamon, nutmeg, and cardamom add the suggestion of sweetness without added sugar. We use them liberally to enhance flavor.

NUTS: Toasting nuts is a small step that pays off when you need to amplify flavor without sugar. Nuts also add texture, which helps round out recipes. For those with allergies, we offer the option to swap seeds for nuts.

DARK CHOCOLATE: With 60 to 63 percent cacao, bittersweet chocolate lends a wonderful richness and depth of flavor to recipes with less sugar than its semisweet counterpart. It's an easy swap.

NUT AND SEED BUTTERS: Peanut, almond, and sunflower seed butters add creamy sweetness with no added sugar. Always choose unsweetened varieties.

WHOLE MILK YOGURT: Full-fat yogurt adds moisture without loading up on saturated fat.

EGG YOLKS: Egg yolks help bind cookies and cakes when using less sugar.

BAKING SODA AND BAKING POWDER: You'll notice that we play around with the amounts of these leaveners in our recipes to achieve the best texture.

GRANULATED SUGAR: White sugar is critical in many recipes, particularly desserts, because it adds structure and sweetness without adding other flavors in the way that honey and maple syrup do. We use it when it's the best ingredient to do the job, but we always keep it to a minimum.

BROWN SUGAR: Brown sugar acts like granulated sugar, but its hint of molasses adds a special touch of flavor that is harder to achieve with granulated sugar. It's key in recipes like Chewy Chocolate Chip Cookies (page 131) and BBQ Sauce (page 185).

HONEY: Honey is a minimally processed sweetener with a range of floral flavors depending on its origin. It has some beneficial properties (see page 5), but it still counts toward your daily added sugar total. Due to its composition, honey has nearly 6 grams of sugar per teaspoon rather than the roughly 4 grams per teaspoon present in granulated sugar. We have accounted for this in our recipes and use it sparingly when we want to highlight its distinctive flavor, as in Honey-Peach Breakfast Pops (page 19).

MAPLE SYRUP: Maple syrup is a less-processed sweetener that adds a unique sweetness and depth of flavor to recipes like Fruit and Nut Granola (page 22) and Caramelized Pumpkin Pie (page 149). Because maple syrup is a common accompaniment with pancakes and waffles, we've created sweet sauces using naturally sweet fruits and a bit of maple syrup that you can use for topping your favorite breakfast treats—Raspberry Sauce (page 38) and Maple Yogurt (page 36). Be sure to choose 100 percent pure maple syrup. Avoid pancake syrups—many contain highly processed ingredients.

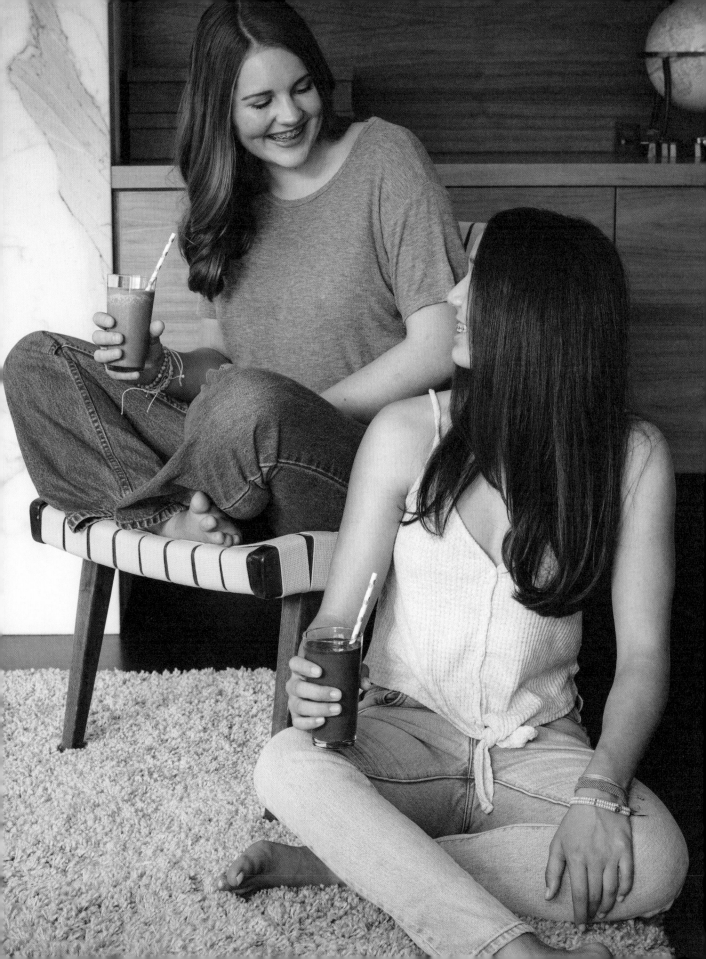

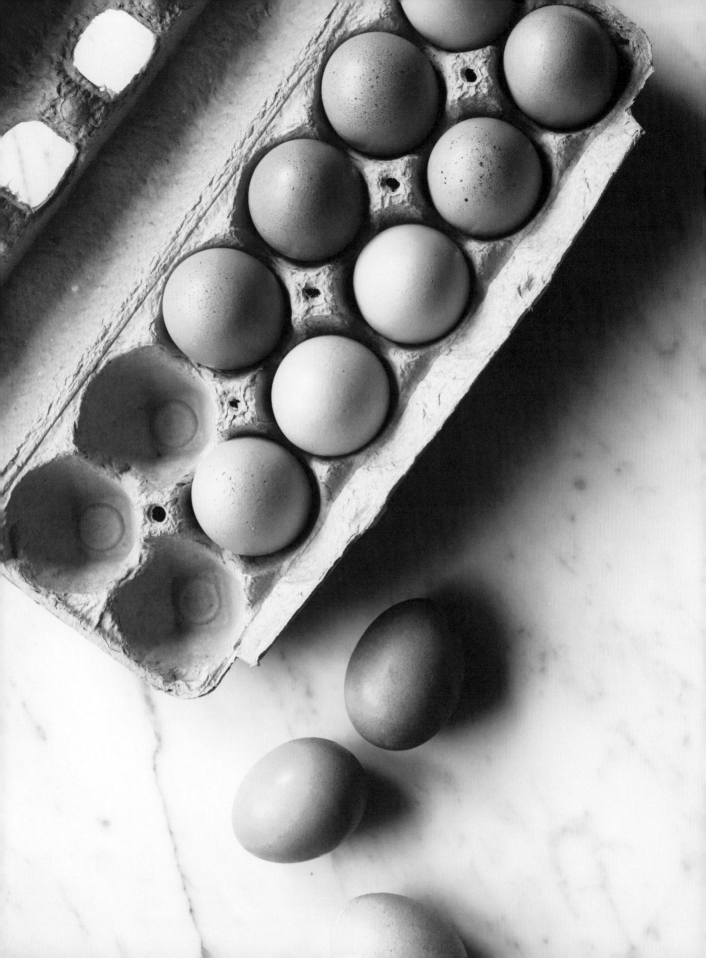

BREAKFASTS

Would you give your child a candy bar for breakfast? The added sugar in a packed-with-peanuts chocolate bar is roughly equivalent to the amount that's hiding in many seemingly healthy breakfast choices, like popular packaged grab-and-go yogurt parfaits. Quick morning solutions such as cold and hot cereals, granola, toaster pastries, and flavored yogurts often contain a tremendous amount of added sugar lurking behind a seemingly healthy label. Happy farm animals, smiling fruits and veggies, and the word "natural" often appear prominently on these products' packaging, which can be deceiving because these items can contain as much sugar as a typical dessert. Similarly, many lazy weekend breakfast treats—like muffins, quick breads, pancakes, and waffles—can easily push you over your daily limit of added sugar in one meal. To reduce added sugar while maximizing flavor, we've remastered weekday and weekend breakfast favorites—from Apple-Cinnamon Instant Oatmeal (page 25) and Honey-Peach Breakfast Pops (page 19) to Pumpkin Spice Waffles (page 35), Super Moist Banana Bread (page 52), and Blueberry-Oat Muffins (page 45)—with naturally sweet fruits and vegetables, making it easy for you and your kids to start the day right.

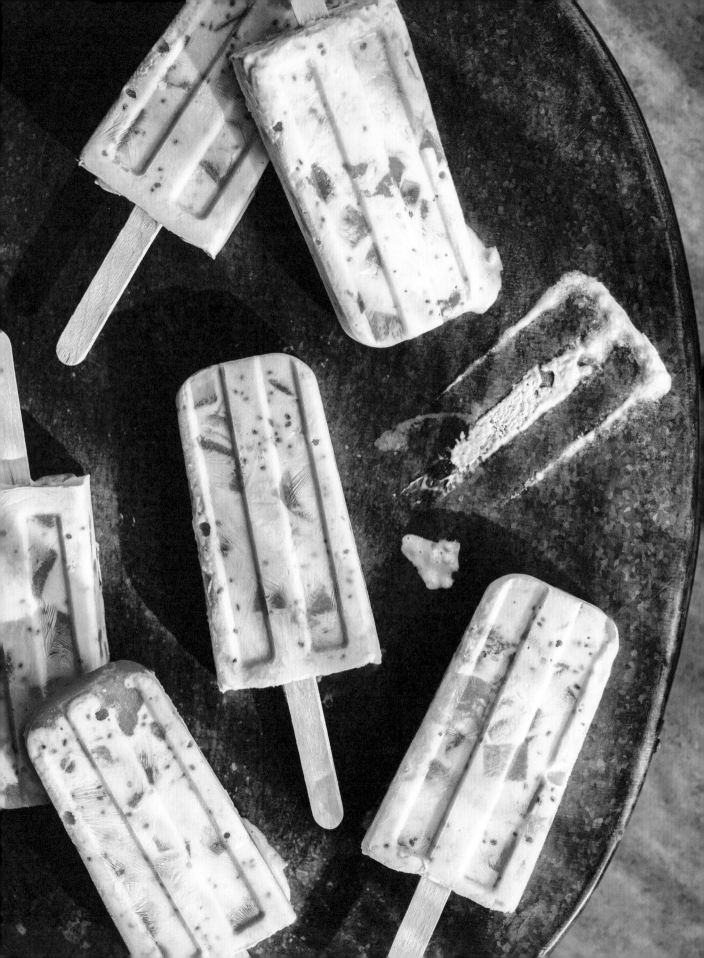

HONEY-PEACH BREAKFAST POPS

OURS = 1¼ TEASPOONS
THEIRS = 3 TO 5 TEASPOONS

These portable breakfast fro-yo pops are perfect for mornings. Naturally sweet peaches and a touch of honey are quickly simmered to bring out even more of their delicious flavor. They are then combined with tangy Greek yogurt and a hint of vanilla to create a creamy pop reminiscent of packaged frozen yogurt with a fraction of the added sugar. Add chia seeds if you'd like a little extra boost of protein. You'll need standard 3-ounce pop molds and sticks for these.

1 Place the peaches, honey, and ¼ cup water in a small saucepan. Bring to a simmer over medium-high heat. Cook, stirring occasionally, until tender and syrupy, about 5 minutes. Transfer to a medium bowl, stir in the vanilla, and let cool completely.

2 Stir the yogurt and chia seeds, if using, into the cooked peaches until combined. Divide among seven 3-ounce ice pop molds. Add sticks and freeze until firm, at least 4 hours.

3 To serve, loosen the pops from the molds by dipping the molds in a bowl of warm water for 15 to 30 seconds.

VARIATION: Use 10 ounces fresh or frozen blueberries or raspberries, or a combo of the two in place of the peaches.

⚡ **QUICK TIP**
Use a 10-ounce bag of unsweetened frozen peaches if you can't find fresh peaches. Thaw and drain before cooking with the honey and water.

☺ **WHAT KIDS CAN DO**
Kids can help pour the mixture into the molds.

☆ **MAKE AHEAD**
The pops will keep in an airtight container in the freezer for up to 1 month.

Ingredients

1 pound ripe peaches (about 3 large fresh peaches), peeled, pitted, and cut into ½-inch chunks

2 tablespoons honey

½ teaspoon pure vanilla extract

1¼ cups whole milk plain Greek yogurt

1 tablespoon chia seeds (optional)

MAKES 7 POPS

NUTRITION INFORMATION (1 POP):
Calories: 83 | Added sugar: 1¼ teaspoons or 5g | Carbohydrates: 13g | Sodium: 14mg | Saturated fat: 11% of calories or 1g | Fiber: 1g | Protein: 4g

CHERRY-OATMEAL BREAKFAST COOKIES

OURS = 1½ TEASPOONS
THEIRS = 3 TEASPOONS

Ingredients

1½ cups old-fashioned (rolled) oats

½ cup all-purpose flour

½ cup whole-wheat pastry flour

1 teaspoon salt

1 teaspoon ground cinnamon

½ teaspoon baking soda

1 large egg plus 1 egg yolk

½ cup mashed very ripe banana (about 1 medium banana)

2 teaspoons pure vanilla extract

1 cup finely grated carrot

½ cup unsweetened dried cherries, chopped

½ cup finely chopped walnuts, sunflower seeds, or pumpkin seeds

¼ cup unsweetened shredded coconut

½ cup (1 stick) unsalted butter, at room temperature

⅔ cup packed dark brown sugar

MAKES 47 SMALL COOKIES

Inspired by the flavors of carrot cake, these chewy oatmeal breakfast cookies are loaded with whole grains, dried fruit, and nuts. This recipe is designed to be flexible, so you can use the types of nuts and fruit you have on hand. Instead of cherries, you can add other chopped dried fruit; just be sure it doesn't contain added sugar. Serve with a glass of milk for a quick and well-rounded breakfast.

1 Line two rimmed baking sheets with parchment paper or silicone baking liners.

2 Combine the oats, all-purpose flour, whole-wheat pastry flour, salt, cinnamon, and baking soda in a medium bowl.

3 Whisk together the egg, egg yolk, banana, and vanilla in another medium bowl. Stir in the carrot, cherries, walnuts, and coconut.

4 Whip the butter and brown sugar in the bowl of a stand mixer on medium-high speed until fluffy and lighter in color, 3 minutes. Scrape the side of the bowl. On low speed, add the flour mixture in three additions, alternating with the carrot mixture in two additions, and mix until just combined.

5 Cover and let sit at room temperature for 30 minutes. Preheat the oven to 350°F.

6 Place 1-tablespoon balls of dough on the prepared baking sheets, 3 inches apart.

7 Bake, one pan at a time, until the cookies are light brown on the bottom and edges and no longer wet on top, 13 to 14 minutes. Let cool on the pan for 2 minutes, then transfer to wire racks to cool completely.

NOTE: Allowing the dough to rest for 30 minutes at room temperature before baking is a tip we learned from Serious Eats. It gives the oats a chance to absorb some of the moisture in the dough, resulting in a crispier cookie.

⚡ **QUICK TIP**
Use ½ cup unsweetened applesauce if you don't have ripe bananas on hand.

☺ **WHAT KIDS CAN DO**
Kids can measure the ingredients, mash the bananas, stir the dough, and portion out the cookies.

☆ **MAKE AHEAD**
You can portion the dough onto a prepared baking sheet, cover, and refrigerate overnight. Or form into balls and freeze overnight or until firm and no longer sticky, then place the balls in a resealable plastic bag and store in the freezer for up to 1 month. To bake, let the dough come to room temperature while you preheat the oven, then bake until the cookies are light brown on the bottom and edges and no longer wet on top, 15 to 17 minutes. The cookies will keep, tightly wrapped in plastic wrap, at room temperature for 2 to 3 days.

NUTRITION INFORMATION (2 COOKIES):
Calories: 143 | Added sugar: 1½ teaspoons or 6g | Carbohydrates: 18g | Sodium: 136mg | Saturated fat: 22% of calories or 3g | Fiber: 2g | Protein: 2g

FRUIT AND NUT GRANOLA

OURS: ½ TEASPOON
THEIRS: 1½ TO 2¼ TEASPOONS

Ingredients

¼ cup maple syrup

¼ cup extra-virgin olive oil

2 teaspoons pure vanilla extract

1 teaspoon ground cinnamon

¼ teaspoon ground nutmeg

¼ teaspoon salt

2 cups old-fashioned (rolled) oats

1 cup whole raw almonds, roughly chopped

½ cup raw walnuts, roughly chopped

½ cup ground flaxseed

½ cup unsweetened shredded coconut

4½ ounces dried apricots (about 1 cup), chopped

MAKES 7 CUPS

Packaged granolas, which seem like a healthy choice, can have more than 2 teaspoons of added sugar per ⅓ cup serving. This remastered recipe has just a fraction of that amount. Dried fruit, nuts, spices, and just a touch of maple syrup add loads of flavor without the need for a lot of sugar. To get those yummy chunks of granola that you're used to, firmly press the mixture into the pan before baking. It's best to make a big batch on a day when you have time to cook, then store it for those days when you need a quick breakfast or snack.

1 Preheat the oven to 300°F. Line a rimmed baking sheet with parchment paper or a silicone baking liner.

2 Whisk together the maple syrup, oil, vanilla, cinnamon, nutmeg, and salt in a large bowl. Add the oats, almonds, walnuts, ground flaxseed, and coconut and stir until evenly coated.

3 Pour the mixture onto the prepared baking sheet. Using an offset spatula or the bottom of a glass, firmly press down on the granola to form an even, compact layer about ½ inch thick. The granola may not cover the entire surface of the baking sheet.

4 Bake the granola for 20 minutes, then rotate the pan 180 degrees and continue baking until golden brown, about 20 minutes more. Let the granola cool completely in the pan, about 1 hour.

5 Gently break the granola into large clumps. Stir in the dried apricots. The granola will continue to break apart into smaller pieces as you stir. Transfer the granola to an airtight container.

VARIATION: Substitute 2 ounces unsweetened dried cherries (about ⅓ cup), chopped, for 2 ounces of the dried apricots.

☺ **WHAT KIDS CAN DO**
Kids can measure and mix the ingredients. They'll also enjoy breaking up the granola into chunks.

☆ **MAKE AHEAD**
The granola will keep in an airtight container at room temperature for up to 2 weeks.

NUTRITION INFORMATION (⅓ CUP):
Calories: 159 | Added sugar: ½ teaspoon or 2g | Carbohydrates: 15g | Sodium: 30mg | Saturated fat: 11% of calories or 2g | Fiber: 3g | Protein: 4g

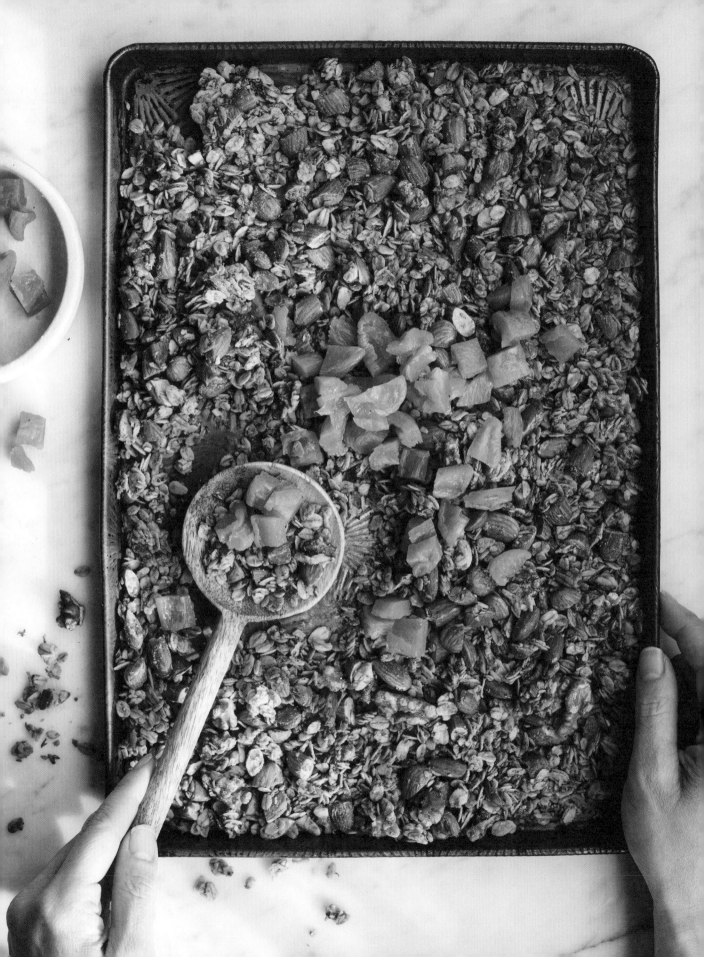

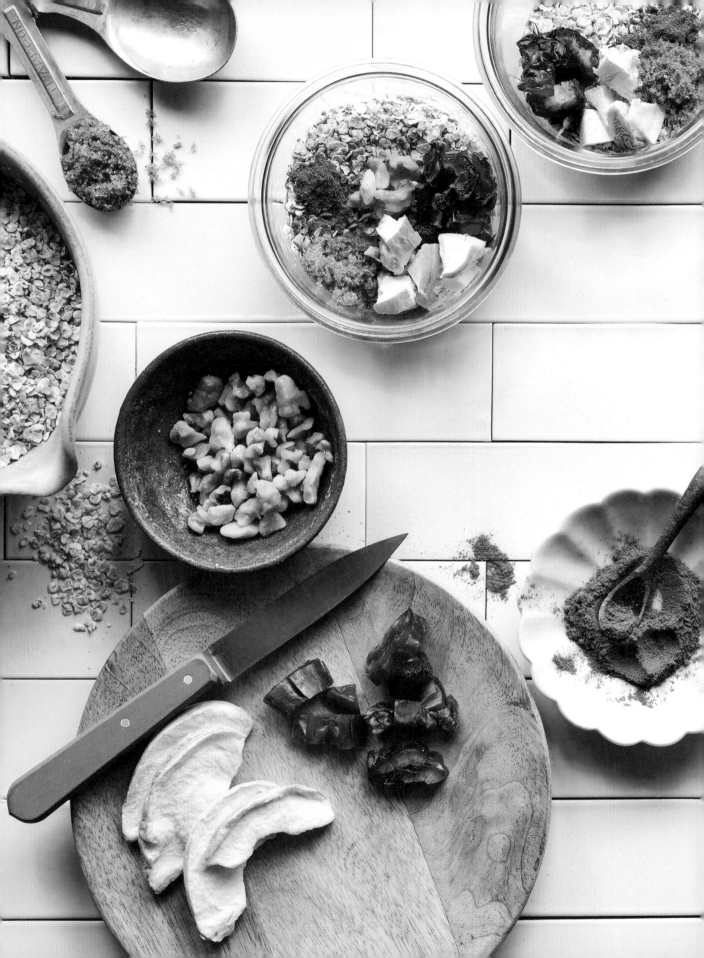

APPLE-CINNAMON INSTANT OATMEAL

OURS = 1 TEASPOON
THEIRS = 2½ TEASPOONS

Freeze-dried apples and dates add natural sweetness, and a dash of cinnamon enhances the flavor of this remastered instant breakfast. Quick oats give the oatmeal a fairly uniform texture, which may be familiar to kids who like the kind from a packet. You'll need twelve wide-mouth heatproof glass containers (12- to 16-ounce size) to hold the oatmeal, which serve as both storage and the serving vessels for this quick breakfast. Just add milk or water to the container, heat it up in the microwave, and breakfast is ready in a few minutes. You can also store individual servings of the oatmeal mixture in small wax paper bags in an airtight container. If you're using bags, you may want a helper to hold them open while you fill them.

TO ASSEMBLE THE INDIVIDUAL SERVINGS:

Spread the glass containers or bags out on the counter and divide the dry ingredients among them as follows: ⅓ cup oats, ½ ounce apples, 1 chopped date, 1 teaspoon brown sugar, ½ teaspoon cinnamon, and a dash of salt. Stir to combine, then cover to store.

TO PREPARE A SERVING IN THE MICROWAVE:

1 Pour the oatmeal mixture into a heatproof bowl (or use the storage jar if it is heatproof), add ⅓ cup water and ⅓ cup milk, and stir well.

2 Heat in the microwave for 2 minutes. Stir again and let sit for 1 minute. Add 1 to 2 tablespoons milk or water, if needed, to achieve desired consistency, and serve immediately.

TO PREPARE A SERVING ON THE STOVETOP:

1 Pour ⅓ cup milk into a small saucepan, add ⅓ cup water, and bring to a simmer over low heat.

2 Place the oatmeal mixture in a heatproof bowl (if not using a heatproof storage jar), add the hot milk mixture, and stir to combine. Let sit 1 minute. Stir again, add 1 to 2 tablespoons milk or water, if needed, to achieve desired consistency, and serve immediately.

Ingredients

4 cups quick-cook oats

6 ounces unsweetened freeze-dried apples, chopped or roughly broken (about 6 cups)

12 Medjool dates (about 10 ounces), pitted and chopped

¼ cup packed light brown sugar

2 tablespoons ground cinnamon

¾ teaspoon salt

Low-fat milk or almond milk, for serving

MAKES 12 SERVINGS

Recipe continues

VARIATIONS: Feel free to mix and match other unsweetened freeze-dried fruits instead of the apples, such as strawberries, bananas, and blueberries, or use unsweetened dried cherries or raisins. Try replacing the brown sugar with maple sugar or coconut sugar. Toasted walnuts, pumpkin seeds, or slivered almonds and fresh fruit make great toppings.

☺ **WHAT KIDS CAN DO**
Kids can help fill the containers.

☆ **MAKE AHEAD**
The instant oatmeal mixture will keep in an airtight container at room temperature for up to 1 month.

NUTRITION INFORMATION (1 SERVING WITH MILK):
Calories: 275 | Added sugar: 1 teaspoon or 4g | Carbohydrates: 59g | Sodium: 209mg | Saturated fat: 3% of calories or 1g | Fiber: 7g | Protein: 7g

STRAWBERRY TOASTER PASTRIES

OURS = ¾ TEASPOON
THEIRS = 3 TO 4 TEASPOONS

Ripe strawberries, lemon juice, and just a touch of sugar make a delicious filling for these kid-friendly toaster pastries. They are best made ahead and then frozen, so you'll have a quick breakfast treat at the ready when time is tight.

1 Make the filling: Place the strawberries in a food processor and pulse to a chunky puree, about 10 pulses. Strain out 2 teaspoons of the strawberry juice.

2 Transfer the strawberries to a small saucepan. Add the granulated sugar and bring to a boil, stirring. Reduce the heat to low and cook, stirring often, until the mixture reduces to a deep red syrup, about 15 minutes.

3 Combine the lemon juice and cornstarch in a small bowl and mix well. Stir into the strawberries, return to a simmer, and cook until thickened, 1 to 2 minutes.

4 Transfer the mixture to a bowl and let cool.

5 When you are ready to form and bake the pastries, preheat the oven to 400°F. Line two baking sheets with parchment paper or silicone baking liners.

6 Make an egg wash: Combine the egg white, confectioners' sugar, and reserved strawberry juice in a small bowl and mix with a fork or whisk until the sugar is dissolved.

7 Divide the pastry dough in half. Flour a work surface and place one disk of the pastry dough on top. Roll it out with a floured rolling pin to an 18 by 10-inch rectangle (or slightly larger) about ⅛ inch thick. Cut the dough into six 3 by 10-inch strips. You will later fold each strip in half to make six 3 x 5-inch tarts.

8 Place 1 level tablespoon of the filling on the bottom half of each strip and spread into a rectangle, leaving a ½-inch border around the edges. Fold the top over, then press the edges together. If any filling gets on the border, just wipe it off to prevent leakage in the oven. Use the tines of a fork to press the edges together firmly to seal, and poke the top of the tart with the fork three times. Repeat with the remaining pastry dough and filling.

9 Brush the top and edges of each toaster pastry with the egg wash.

Recipe continues

Ingredients

1 pint strawberries, hulled (12 ounces), or 8 ounces unsweetened frozen strawberries (about 2 cups), thawed
2 tablespoons granulated sugar
1 tablespoon freshly squeezed lemon juice or water
1 tablespoon cornstarch
2 tablespoons egg white
2 tablespoons confectioners' sugar
All-purpose flour, for dusting
1 recipe Pastry Dough (page 203)

MAKES 12 PASTRIES

10 Place the pastries on the prepared baking sheets and bake until the tops and edges are golden, 13 to 15 minutes.

11 To serve, let cool on the baking sheets for 10 minutes, then transfer to a wire rack to cool longer before serving. Be careful because the filling is hot!

⚡ **QUICK TIP**
Use two flat frozen pie crusts (preferably ones with no added sugar; 11 ounces each), thawed according to the package directions. Roll out into rectangles and cut as specified.

☺ **WHAT KIDS CAN DO**
Use a fork to press the edges of the pastries together.

☆ **MAKE AHEAD**
The filling can be made 2 days ahead, covered tightly, and refrigerated. The cooled pastries will keep, tightly wrapped in plastic wrap, in the refrigerator for up to 3 days or in the freezer for up to 1 month. To reheat, unwrap and warm in a 350°F oven for 15 minutes. Leave on the pan for 10 minutes to finish crisping up, then serve.

NUTRITION INFORMATION (1 PASTRY):
Calories: 235 | Added sugar: ¾ teaspoon or 3g | Carbohydrates: 22g | Sodium: 201mg | Saturated fat: 37% of calories or 10g | Fiber: 1g | Protein: 3g

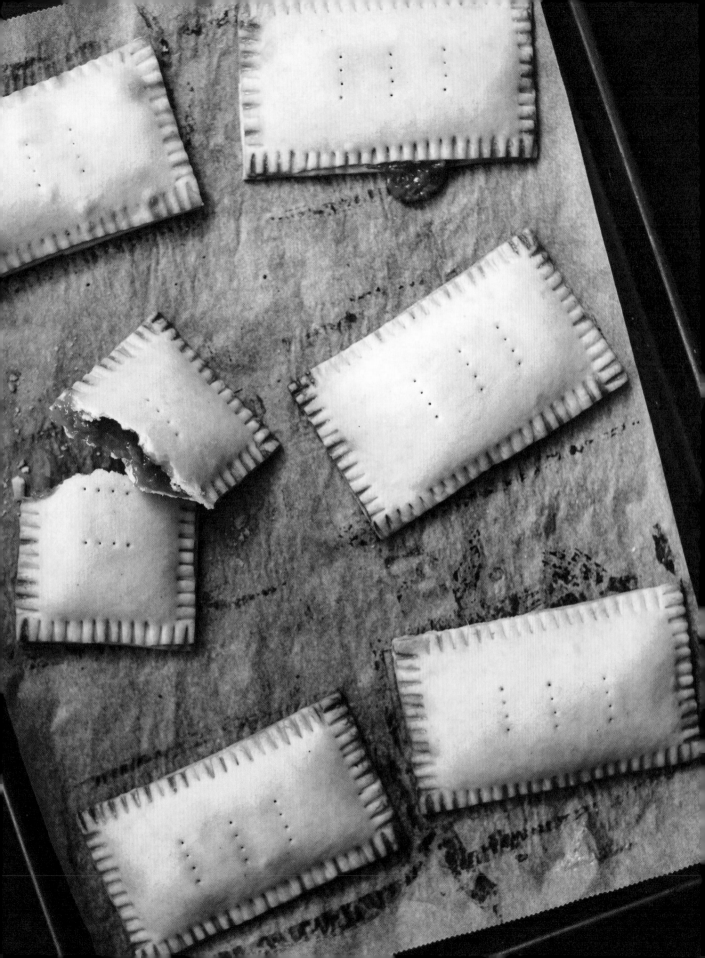

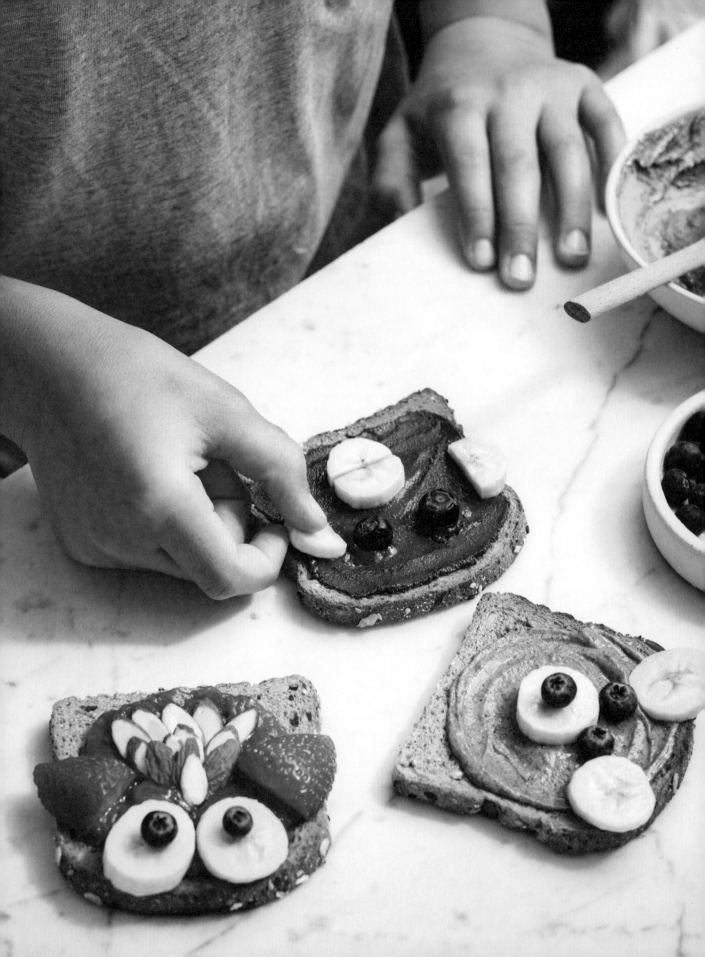

MONKEY TOAST

OURS = ¾ TEASPOON
THEIRS = 2¾ TEASPOONS

Homemade chocolate hazelnut spread, a few slices of banana, and a pop of blueberries make a quick and fun breakfast. Let your kids monkey around to come up with their own fun faces.

1 Toast the bread in a toaster or oven until golden brown, about 2 minutes.

2 Spread the Newtella evenly on one side of the toast. Place the banana slices on the bread to create the two ears and mouth. Add blueberries for the eyes. Serve immediately.

☺ **WHAT KIDS CAN DO**
Little chefs can decorate their own toast.

NUTRITION INFORMATION (1 TOAST):
Calories: 186 | Added sugar: ¾ teaspoon or 3g | Carbohydrates: 19g | Sodium: 182mg | Saturated fat: 8% of calories or 2g | Fiber: 4g | Protein: 6g

Ingredients

1 slice whole-wheat sandwich bread
1 tablespoon Newtella (page 196) or Nut-Free Newtella (page 197)
2 banana slices, cut in half to make four semicircles
2 fresh blueberries

SERVES 1

OWL TOAST

OURS = ½ TEASPOON
THEIRS = 2¾ TEASPOONS

Ingredients

1 slice whole-wheat
    sandwich bread
1 tablespoon Three-
    Ingredient Strawberry
    Jam (page 198)
2 banana slices
2 fresh blueberries
About 12 almond slices
1 whole almond (optional)
1 large strawberry, hulled
    and halved lengthwise
    (to form 2 wing-shaped
    pieces)

SERVES 1

Toast with jam is more fun when it's dressed up as a friendly owl. Here our simple homemade low-sugar jam is combined with sliced almonds, bananas, and blueberries to create a woodland animal sweet enough to eat.

1 Toast the bread in a toaster or oven until golden brown, about 2 minutes.

2 Spread the strawberry jam evenly on one side of the toast. Place 2 banana slices on the toast and top with the blueberries to create the eyes. Starting from the bottom, layer most of the sliced almonds in rows to create the feathers (reserve one if you are not using the whole almond for the beak). Add the whole almond or reserved almond slice for the beak and the strawberry slices for the wings. Serve immediately.

NUTRITION INFORMATION (1 TOAST):
Calories: 134 | Added sugar: ½ teaspoon or 2g | Carbohydrates: 20g | Sodium: 133mg | Saturated fat: 3% of calories or <1g | Fiber: 4g | Protein: 5g

BEAR TOAST

 OURS = ¼ TEASPOON
THEIRS = ¾ TEASPOON

Perfect for a teddy bear's picnic, this quick and easy breakfast toast combines naturally sweet peanut butter, bananas, and blueberries. If your little bears are like ours, they'll love this as an after-school snack, too.

1 Toast the bread in a toaster or oven until golden brown, about 2 minutes.

2 Spread the nut butter evenly on one side of the toast. Place the banana slices on the toast to create the ears and snout. Add 2 blueberries for the eyes and 1 blueberry for the tip of the nose. Serve immediately.

NUTRITION INFORMATION (1 TOAST):
Calories: 188 | Added sugar: ¼ teaspoon or 1g | Carbohydrates: 20g | Sodium: 132mg | Saturated fat: 7% of calories or 1g | Fiber: 4g | Protein: 8g

Ingredients

1 slice whole-wheat sandwich bread
1 tablespoon unsweetened peanut butter, unsweetened sunflower seed butter, or unsweetened almond butter
3 banana slices
3 fresh blueberries

SERVES 1

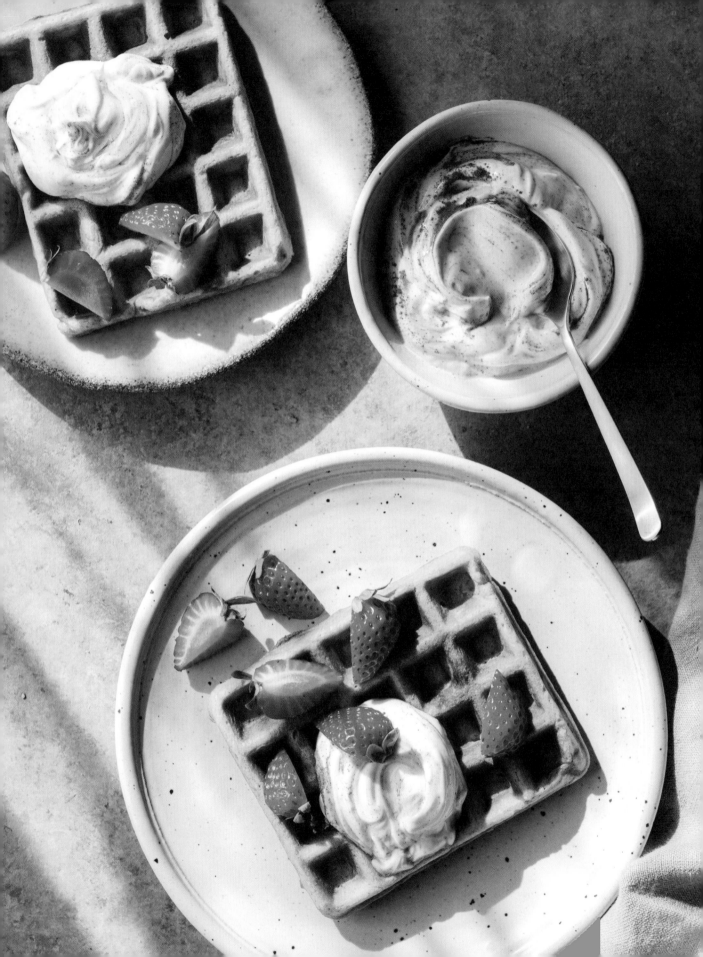

PUMPKIN SPICE WAFFLES
WITH MAPLE YOGURT

OURS = 1½ TEASPOONS
THEIRS = 15 TO 16 TEASPOONS

Pumpkin puree adds delicious fall flavor, natural sweetness, and a boost of vegetables to these classic waffles. A touch of brown sugar adds crispness. Loads of maple syrup is the real culprit with waffles and pancakes, so to slash the added sugar, serve up these waffles with Maple Yogurt (page 36) and fresh fruit. If you'd like to add some protein, sprinkle finely chopped pecans or walnuts on top of the batter after you pour it into the waffle maker. You can also serve these waffles with a dollop of Maple-Vanilla Whipped Cream (page 199), if you prefer. This recipe makes a big batch, but luckily these waffles freeze well, making them a quick breakfast on busy mornings.

1 Preheat a waffle maker to medium heat.

2 Combine the flour, brown sugar, baking powder, cinnamon, ginger, salt, and nutmeg in a large bowl.

3 Whisk together the milk, oil, butter, vanilla, eggs, and pumpkin puree in a medium bowl. Whisk the wet ingredients into the dry ingredients until just combined.

4 Add about ½ cup batter (or the amount called for in your waffle maker instructions) to the waffle maker and spread out with a silicone spatula. Cook for 1 to 2 minutes longer than indicated on the machine because the pumpkin makes the batter denser so it takes longer to cook. You can check if the waffles are cooked through by tearing off a corner.

5 Serve the waffles right away, with the Maple Yogurt, and fresh fruit on the side, if using.

NOTE: Be sure to use canned unsweetened pumpkin puree here, *not* pumpkin pie filling.

☺ **WHAT KIDS CAN DO**
Little chefs can whisk together the Maple Yogurt. Older kids can toast their own frozen waffles.

Recipe continues

Ingredients

3 cups all-purpose flour
¼ cup packed light brown sugar
4 teaspoons baking powder
2 teaspoons ground cinnamon
2 teaspoons ground ginger
1 teaspoon salt
⅛ teaspoon ground nutmeg or ground allspice
2 cups low-fat milk
½ cup canola oil
½ cup (1 stick) unsalted butter, melted and cooled
4 teaspoons pure vanilla extract
4 large eggs
1 can (15 ounces) pumpkin puree (about 2 cups; see Note)
Maple Yogurt (page 36), for serving
2 to 4 cups fresh blueberries, raspberries, sliced strawberries, peaches, apricots, bananas, or other fresh fruit, for serving (optional)

MAKES 14 LARGE WAFFLES

★ **MAKE AHEAD**
To prep the batter the night before, mix together the dry ingredients in a large bowl and the wet ingredients (except for the melted butter) in another bowl, then cover with plastic wrap and refrigerate the wet mixture. Keep the wet ingredients separated from the dry ingredients so that the baking powder stays active; otherwise you'll have flat, dense waffles. In the morning, combine the two and add the melted butter.

To make frozen waffles, cook the waffles in your waffle maker until they are lightly golden brown on the outside but still soft in the middle, 3 to 4 minutes for a large waffle or roughly three-fourths of the total cooking time on your machine. Set them on a wire rack to cool completely.

The waffles will keep, tightly wrapped in plastic wrap, in the freezer for up to a month. To reheat, unwrap the waffles, let them thaw, then place them on a baking sheet and bake in a 375°F oven until they are warmed through and golden brown, about 10 minutes. Or you can pop the thawed waffles into the toaster.

NUTRITION INFORMATION (1 LARGE WAFFLE WITH 2 TABLESPOONS MAPLE YOGURT):
Calories: 326 | Added sugar: 1½ teaspoons or 6g | Carbohydrates: 34g | Sodium: 219mg | Saturated fat: 16% of calories or 6g | Fiber: 2g | Protein: 9g

Maple Yogurt

OURS = ¾ TEASPOON
THEIRS = 12 TEASPOONS

Ingredients

2 cups low-fat plain Greek yogurt
3 tablespoons maple syrup
½ teaspoon ground cinnamon

MAKES ABOUT 2 CUPS

Whisk together the yogurt, maple syrup, and cinnamon in a serving bowl.

★ **MAKE AHEAD**
The yogurt will keep in an airtight container in the refrigerator for up to 1 week.

NUTRITION INFORMATION (ABOUT 2 TABLESPOONS):
Calories: 35 | Added sugar: ¾ teaspoon or 3g | Carbohydrates: 4g | Sodium: 11mg | Saturated fat: 10% of calories or <1g | Fiber: 0g | Protein: 3g

OVERNIGHT FRENCH TOAST STRATA
WITH RASPBERRY SAUCE

◼◻◻◻◻◻◻◻◻◻◻◻◻◻◻◻◻ OURS: 1 TEASPOON
THEIRS: 15 TO 16 TEASPOONS

Ripe banana adds natural sweetness to this easy French toast strata. A sweet and tangy raspberry sauce satisfies your cravings for a syrupy topping without all that sugar. Both the sauce and the strata can be made ahead, making this a perfect recipe for when you're hosting a special weekend brunch with friends and family.

1 Butter the bottom and sides of a 13 × 9-inch baking dish. Arrange the challah cubes evenly in the pan in a snug, single layer.

2 Peel the banana, break it into quarters, and place it in a blender. Add the milk, vanilla, cinnamon, salt, nutmeg, and eggs. Cover and blend until smooth, about 1 minute. Pour the mixture over the bread, pressing down the cubes with the back of a spoon to ensure that they are fully covered with the custard. Cover with aluminum foil and refrigerate overnight or for up to 12 hours.

3 Preheat the oven to 375°F.

4 Place the pan on a rimmed baking sheet, leaving the foil on. Bake, covered, for 30 minutes. Remove the foil and continue baking until the challah has puffed and is evenly browned, 25 to 30 minutes more.

5 Cut the strata into 8 pieces and serve topped with the raspberry sauce and fresh berries.

☺ **WHAT KIDS CAN DO**
With clean hands or the back of a spoon, kids can gently press down the bread cubes to make sure they are fully soaked in the custard.

☆ **MAKE AHEAD**
The French toast strata should be assembled and refrigerated the night before. The raspberry sauce can be made the night before (see recipe) Warm it before serving.

Ingredients

1 tablespoon unsalted butter, at room temperature
1 loaf (1 pound) challah bread, preferably day-old, cut into 1-inch cubes
1 ripe medium banana
3 cups whole milk
2 teaspoons pure vanilla extract
1 teaspoon ground cinnamon
½ teaspoon salt
⅛ teaspoon ground nutmeg
4 large eggs
Raspberry Sauce (page 38), for serving
1 cup fresh raspberries, for serving

SERVES 8

NUTRITION INFORMATION (1 PIECE WITH 2½ TABLESPOONS SAUCE):
Calories: 325 | Added sugar: 1 teaspoon or 4g | Carbohydrates: 46g | Sodium: 500mg | Saturated fat: 12% of calories or 4g | Fiber: 6g | Protein: 12g

Raspberry Sauce

OURS = ¾ TEASPOON
THEIRS = 12 TEASPOONS

Ingredients

12 ounces (about 2¾ cups)
   fresh raspberries
2 tablespoons maple syrup

MAKES 1¼ CUPS

Combine the raspberries and
maple syrup in a small saucepan
over medium-high heat. Cook,
stirring occasionally, until the
raspberries have broken down
and the mixture is syrupy, about
10 minutes.

⭐ **MAKE AHEAD**
The rasperry sauce will keep
in an airtight container in the
refrigerator for 1 day.

NUTRITION INFORMATION (2½ TABLESPOONS):
Calories: 35 | Added sugar: ¾ teaspoon or 3g | Carbohydrates: 8g | Sodium: 1mg |
Saturated fat: 0% of calories or 0g | Fiber: 3g | Protein: 1g

BLUEBERRY SCONES

 OURS = ¾ TEASPOON
THEIRS: 2¼ TEASPOONS

These homemade scones have just a fraction of the added sugar found in most coffee shop–style scones, thanks to the help of pear puree and plenty of fresh blueberries. To cut down on the amount of saturated fat in each of these breakfast treats, whole milk yogurt stands in for heavy cream. A touch of lemon zest adds brightness.

1 Preheat the oven to 450°F. Line a rimmed baking sheet with parchment paper.

2 Place 2 cups of the flour, the sugar, baking powder, lemon zest, and salt in a food processor. Pulse until combined, about 10 pulses. Add the butter and pulse until the mixture is crumbly, about 20 pulses. Transfer the mixture to a large bowl.

3 Place the pear and yogurt in the now-empty food processor and process until smooth, stopping to scrape down the side of the bowl as needed, 1 to 2 minutes. Add the egg and pulse to combine, about 10 pulses.

4 Pour the yogurt mixture over the flour mixture and stir until just combined. Carefully fold in the blueberries, using your hands if needed to help incorporate the berries into the dough.

5 Place the dough on a lightly floured work surface and dust the top lightly with 2 tablespoons of flour. Pat the dough into an 8-inch circle, about 1 inch thick. Cut into 8 even wedges. Transfer the scones to the prepared baking sheet, spacing them evenly apart.

6 Bake until the scones are golden brown on the top and bottom, 20 to 22 minutes, rotating the baking sheet 180 degrees halfway through baking.

7 Let the scones cool for 5 minutes before transferring to a wire rack. Let cool for at least 10 minutes before serving.

VARIATIONS: In lieu of blueberries and lemon zest, try 1½ cups diced peaches with ½ teaspoon ground ginger and/or almond extract, 1½ cups blackberries with 1 tablespoon lime zest, or 1½ cups chopped strawberries with 1 teaspoon pure vanilla extract (with or without the lemon zest).

Recipe continues

Ingredients

2 cups all-purpose flour, plus extra for dusting
2 tablespoons sugar
1 tablespoon baking powder
1 tablespoon finely grated lemon zest
½ teaspoon salt
6 tablespoons (¾ stick) cold unsalted butter, cut into 6 pieces
½ ripe d'Anjou pear, cored and coarsely chopped (about 4 ounces)
½ cup whole milk plain yogurt
1 large egg
1½ cups fresh blueberries

MAKES 8 SCONES

⚡ **QUICK TIP**
Substitute ¼ cup unsweetened
applesauce for the pear and proceed
as directed.

☺ **WHAT KIDS CAN DO**
Little chefs can fold in the
blueberries.

☆ **MAKE AHEAD**
The scones will keep in an airtight
container at room temperature for
up to 3 days. For the best flavor,
warm in a 350°F oven for 5 to 7
minutes. Let cool for 5 minutes
before serving.

NUTRITION INFORMATION (1 SCONE):
Calories: 246 | Added sugar: ¾ teaspoon or 3g | Carbohydrates: 35g | Sodium: 165mg |
Saturated fat: 22% of calories or 6g | Fiber: 2g | Protein: 5g

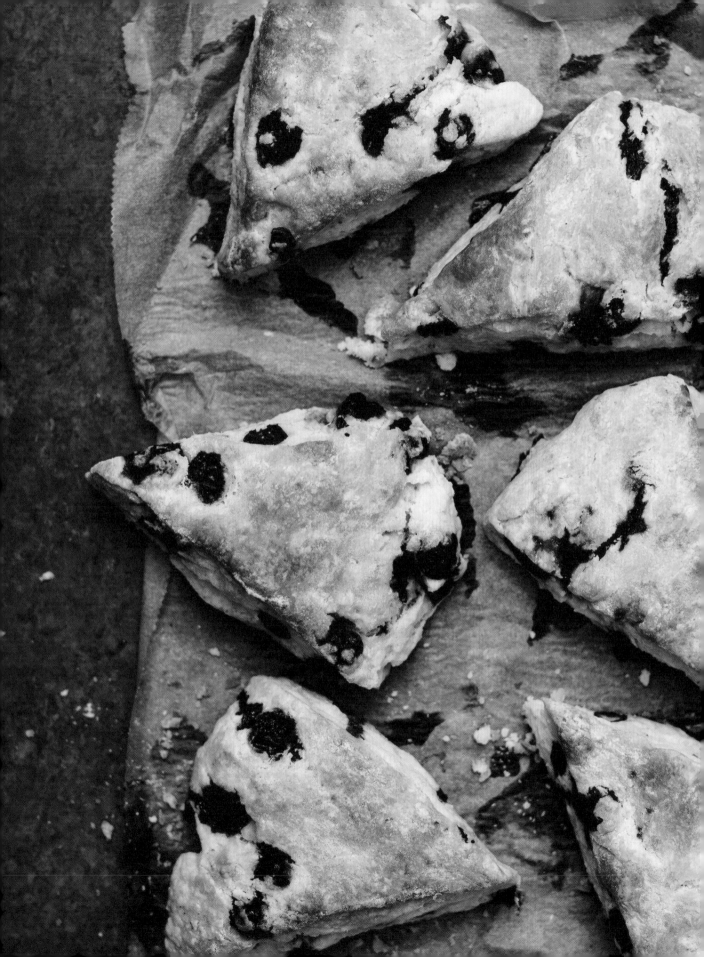

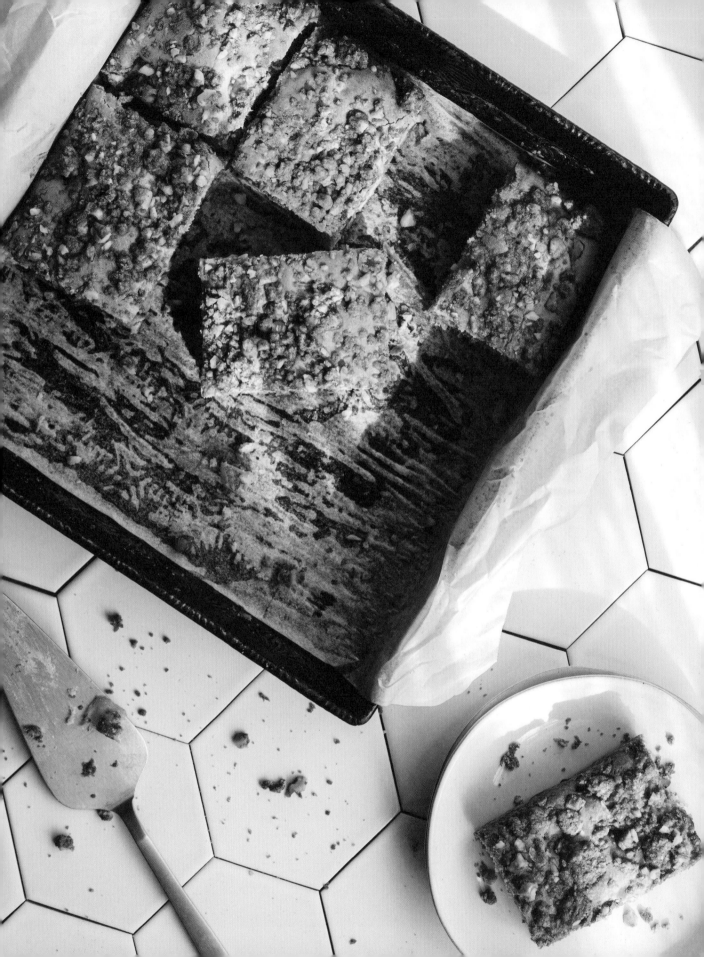

CINNAMON-APPLE COFFEE CAKE

OURS = 3¼ TEASPOONS
THEIRS = 6½ TEASPOONS

Cinnamon-spiced apples add loads of sweet, fruity flavor to this classic coffee cake. The topping, which also doubles as a delicious streusel-style layer, combines walnuts, brown sugar, and cinnamon in just the right proportions to round out the flavors. Cakes and quick breads with less sugar can be dry, so this recipe uses yogurt and an extra egg yolk to ensure a tender crumb. You'll be hard pressed to have just one piece.

1 Preheat the oven to 350°F and line an 8-inch square pan with parchment paper, leaving 2 inches of overhang on each side. Coat the paper with cooking spray.

2 Make the crumble: Place the walnuts, flour, brown sugar, cinnamon, and salt in a food processor and process until the nuts are finely chopped, 30 seconds to 1 minute. Add the butter and pulse until you get a clumpy mixture, 10 to 15 pulses.

3 Make the cake: Combine 1 tablespoon of the flour with ½ teaspoon of the cinnamon in a small bowl. Add the apple pieces and stir to coat. Set aside.

4 In a large bowl, combine the remaining 2 cups flour, 1 teaspoon cinnamon, the baking powder, baking soda, and salt. Whisk to combine.

5 Combine the melted butter with the granulated sugar in the bowl of a stand mixer fitted with a paddle attachment. Beat for 1 minute. Add the eggs, egg yolk, and vanilla and beat until combined, about 30 seconds. With the mixer on low, add the flour mixture in three additions, alternating with the yogurt or sour cream. Increase the speed to medium and beat until no flour is visible, about 30 seconds more. Scrape down the bowl, add the milk, and mix until just combined. Stir in the apple mixture.

6 Transfer half of the cake batter to the prepared pan, spreading it evenly all the way to the sides in a thin layer. Add half of the crumble, sprinkling it with your fingers and leaving a border around the edges. Repeat with the remaining cake batter, making sure to spread it all the way to the edges, and top with the remaining crumble.

Recipe continues

Ingredients

Nonstick cooking spray

FOR THE CRUMBLE
½ cup chopped walnuts
⅓ cup all-purpose flour
¼ cup packed dark brown sugar
2 teaspoons ground cinnamon
¼ teaspoon salt
4 tablespoons (½ stick) cold unsalted butter, cut into pieces

FOR THE CAKE
2 cups plus 1 tablespoon all-purpose flour
1½ teaspoons ground cinnamon
1 Granny Smith apple, peeled, cored, and cut into ½-inch pieces
½ teaspoon baking powder
½ teaspoon baking soda
¼ teaspoon salt
½ cup (1 stick) unsalted butter, melted and cooled
½ cup granulated sugar
2 large eggs plus 1 large egg yolk
2 teaspoons pure vanilla extract
1 cup whole milk plain yogurt or sour cream
¼ cup whole milk

SERVES 12

7 Bake until a toothpick inserted in the center comes out clean, about 55 minutes. Let cool in the pan for at least 15 minutes, then cut into 12 pieces before serving.

WHAT KIDS CAN DO
Kids can sprinkle on the crumble topping.

MAKE AHEAD
The cake will keep, tightly wrapped in plastic wrap, in the refrigerator for up to 3 days.

NUTRITION INFORMATION (1 PIECE):
Calories: 319 | Added sugar: 3¼ teaspoons or 13g | Carbohydrates: 37g | Sodium: 177mg | Saturated fat: 24% or 8g | Fiber: 2g | Protein: 6g

BLUEBERRY-OAT MUFFINS ⬡

OURS: 0 TEASPOONS
THEIRS: 2 TO 5 TEASPOONS

These hearty blueberry muffins are chock-full of naturally sweet blueberries and wholesome grains, making them great for breakfast or a midday snack. The secret ingredient used to sweeten them is dates, resulting in a moist muffin with a lovely crumb, just enough sweetness, and zero added sugar. Lemon zest adds brightness and rounds out the flavor, so be sure to include it. These blueberry muffins do not taste like the fluffy, cupcake-like, white-flour muffins you'd find at a bakery—if you'd like to add a little more sweetness, slice the muffins and drizzle them with a touch of honey or add a small dollop of Three-Ingredient Strawberry Jam (page 198).

Ingredients

Nonstick cooking spray
10 ounces Medjool dates, pitted (about 12 dates)
2 cups hot water
2 cups old-fashioned (rolled) oats
1 cup whole-wheat flour
½ cup ground flaxseed
2 teaspoons baking powder
1 teaspoon ground cinnamon
¾ teaspoon salt
½ teaspoon baking soda
1 cup whole milk plain Greek yogurt
¾ cup canola oil
1 tablespoon pure vanilla extract
2 teaspoons finely grated lemon zest
1 large egg
7½ ounces blueberries (about 1½ cups)

MAKES 12 MUFFINS

1 Preheat the oven to 375°F. Coat a 12-cup muffin pan with cooking spray or line with paper liners.

2 Place the pitted dates in a medium bowl. Cover the dates with the hot water. Set aside until the dates are softened, 10 minutes. Drain the dates, reserving ½ cup of the soaking liquid.

3 Place the oats in a food processor and process until powdery, 1 to 2 minutes. Transfer to a large bowl. Add the flour, flaxseed, baking powder, cinnamon, salt, and baking soda and whisk until combined.

4 Place the dates, ½ cup reserved soaking liquid, the yogurt, oil, vanilla, lemon zest, and egg in the food processor and process until smooth and no flecks of dates remain, about 2 minutes.

5 Pour the yogurt mixture over the flour mixture and stir until just combined. Fold in the blueberries.

6 Divide the batter evenly among the prepared wells of the muffin pan. Bake until the tops are golden brown and a toothpick inserted in the center of a muffin comes out clean, 22 to 24 minutes, rotating the pan 180 degrees halfway through baking.

Recipe continues

7 Let the muffins cool in the pan for 10 minutes. Transfer to a wire rack and let cool for at least 20 minutes before serving.

☺ WHAT KIDS CAN DO

Kids can measure and stir the ingredients and scoop the batter into the wells of the muffin pan.

☆ MAKE AHEAD

The muffins are best eaten the day they are made but will keep in an airtight container at room temperature for up to 2 days, or in a resealable plastic bag in the freezer for up to 1 month. Thaw as needed. For the best flavor, warm in a 375°F oven for 5 to 10 minutes before serving.

NUTRITION INFORMATION (1 MUFFIN):
Calories: 333 | Added sugar: 0 teaspoons or 0g | Carbohydrates: 40g | Sodium: 213mg | Saturated fat: 5% of calories or 2g | Fiber: 6g | Protein: 7g

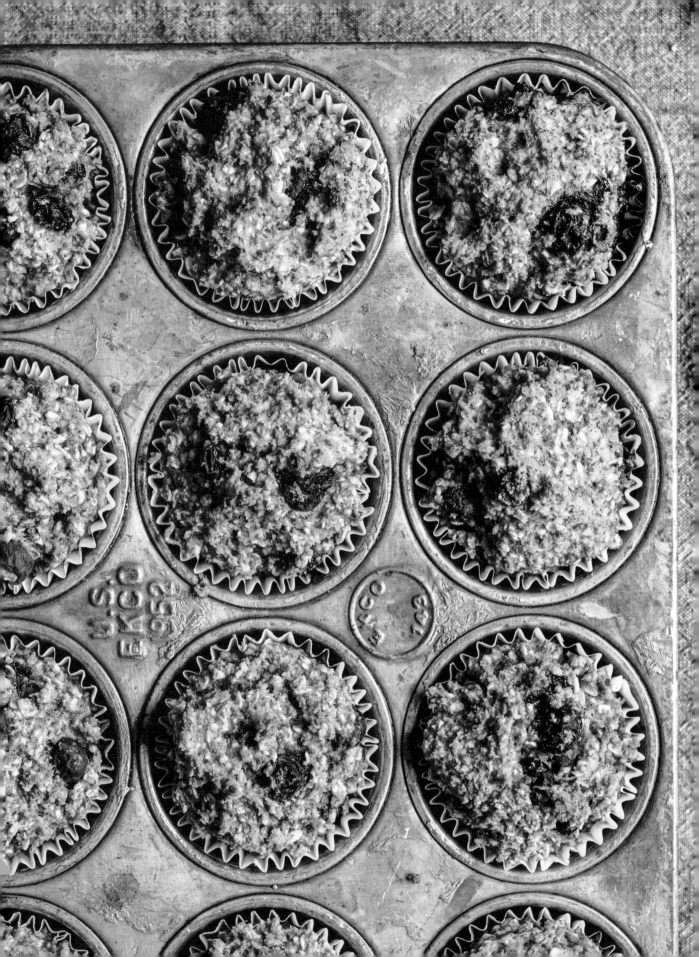

BANANA-CHOCOLATE MUFFINS

OURS = 1¾ TEASPOONS
THEIRS = 3¾ TEASPOONS

Ingredients

Nonstick cooking spray
1½ cups all-purpose flour
¼ cup packed light brown sugar
2 tablespoons unsweetened natural cocoa powder
1 teaspoon baking powder
½ teaspoon baking soda
½ teaspoon salt
3 ounces bittersweet chocolate chips (about ½ cup)
1½ cups mashed very ripe bananas (3 to 4 medium bananas)
¾ cup low-fat milk
4 tablespoons (½ stick) unsalted butter, melted and cooled
1 teaspoon pure vanilla extract
1 large egg
½ cup chopped walnuts or pecans (optional)

MAKES 12 MUFFINS

A cozy batch of banana muffins makes a delicious breakfast or after-school snack. Super-ripe bananas are the stars of the show here. The trick is using dark, speckled ones. That ensures that the natural sugars have had time to develop, which will really shine through in this recipe. The addition of unsweetened cocoa powder and melted bittersweet chocolate adds depth and flavor without too much added sugar. For texture, you can add chopped walnuts or pecans if you choose.

1 Preheat the oven to 375°F. Coat a 12-cup muffin pan with cooking spray or line with paper liners.

2 Combine the flour, brown sugar, cocoa powder, baking powder, baking soda, and salt in a medium bowl.

3 Melt 1 ounce of the chocolate chips in the microwave, stirring at 30-second intervals until almost fully melted, about 1½ minutes total (the chocolate will continue melting as it sits). Let cool briefly.

4 Whisk together the bananas, milk, butter, vanilla, egg, and melted chocolate in a large bowl. Slowly fold in the flour mixture until incorporated, then fold in the remaining 2 ounces chocolate chips and the chopped nuts, if using. The mixture will be thick.

5 Divide the batter evenly among the prepared wells of the muffin pan. Bake until the tops bounce back when you touch them and a toothpick inserted in the center of a muffin comes out clean, 20 to 22 minutes, rotating the pan 180 degrees halfway through baking.

6 Let cool for 10 minutes in the pan, then serve. These muffins are best eaten the day they are made.

QUICK TIP

If you're using walnuts, they will be even more flavorful if you toast them before baking. Place the walnuts on a rimmed baking sheet and bake in the preheated oven until lightly toasted, about 5 minutes. Transfer to a cutting board and let cool before adding to the batter in Step 4.

WHAT KIDS CAN DO

Kids can mash the bananas and portion the batter into the muffin pan.

MAKE AHEAD

The muffins will keep, tightly wrapped in plastic wrap, at room temperature for up to 3 days, or in a resealable plastic bag in the freezer for up to 1 month. Thaw as needed. For the best flavor, warm in a 375°F oven for 5 to 10 minutes before serving.

NUTRITION INFORMATION (1 MUFFIN):
Calories: 190 | Added sugar: 1¾ teaspoons or 7g | Carbohydrates: 28g | Sodium: 166mg | Saturated fat: 20% of calories or 4g | Fiber: 2g | Protein: 4g

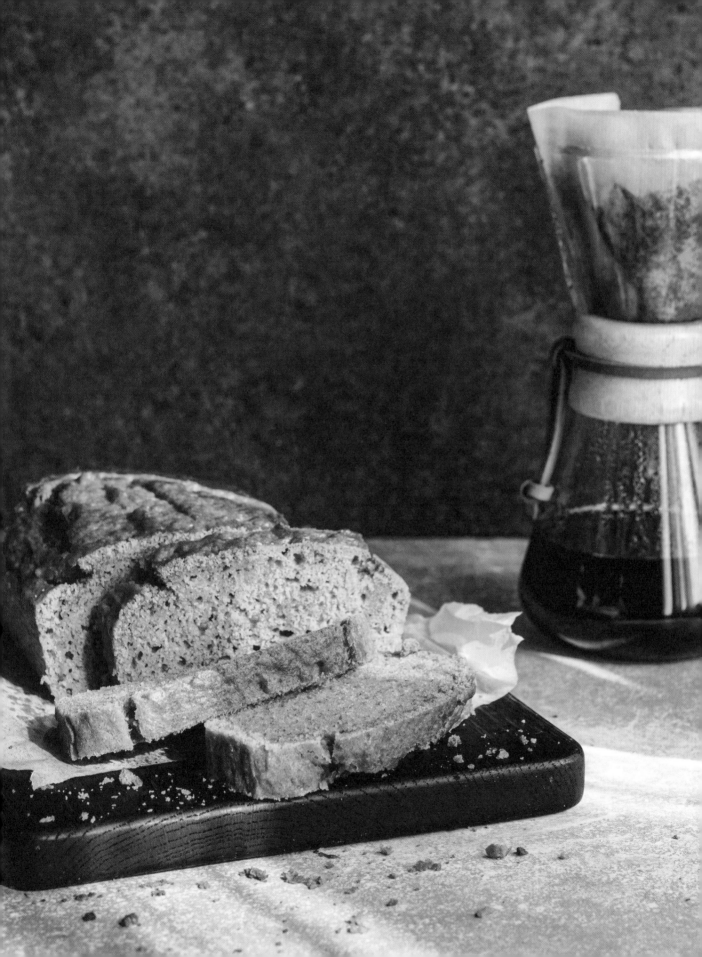

CARAMELIZED PUMPKIN BREAD

OURS = 1½ TEASPOONS
THEIRS = 3½ TO 5¼ TEASPOONS

A warm slice of pumpkin bread is a quintessential fall treat. The smell of it baking makes the whole house feel inviting. Coffee shop–style pumpkin bread can have over 5 teaspoons of added sugar per serving. Caramelizing the pumpkin and banana with a little maple syrup brings out their natural sweetness and enhances the delicious fall flavors with considerably less added sugar. Greek yogurt adds a bit of tang.

1 Preheat the oven to 350°F. Line an 8½ × 4½-inch loaf pan with parchment paper, leaving about 2 inches of overhang on each side. Coat with cooking spray.

2 In a large bowl, whisk together the flour, cinnamon, baking powder, ginger, baking soda, salt, nutmeg, and cloves. Set aside.

3 Combine the pumpkin puree and mashed banana with the maple syrup in a medium saucepan over medium heat. Cook, stirring frequently, until slightly darkened and caramelized, 5 to 7 minutes. Transfer to another large bowl and let cool completely, 15 minutes.

4 Add the oil, yogurt, vanilla, and eggs to the cooled pumpkin mixture and whisk vigorously to combine.

5 Add the flour mixture to the pumpkin mixture and stir gently to combine. (The batter will be thick.)

6 Pour the batter into the prepared loaf pan. Bake until a toothpick inserted into the center comes out clean, 55 minutes to 1 hour.

7 Cool in the pan for 20 minutes, then remove the bread from the pan and transfer to a wire rack. Let cool for at least 15 minutes longer before cutting into 10 slices and serving.

☺ **WHAT KIDS CAN DO**
Kids can mash the banana.

☆ **MAKE AHEAD**
The bread will keep, tightly wrapped in plastic wrap, in the refrigerator for up to 3 days or in the freezer for up to 1 month.

Ingredients

Nonstick cooking spray
1¾ cups all-purpose flour
2 teaspoons ground cinnamon
1½ teaspoons baking powder
1 teaspoon ground ginger
½ teaspoon baking soda
½ teaspoon salt
½ teaspoon ground nutmeg
¼ teaspoon ground cloves
1 cup canned pumpkin puree (see Note, page 35)
½ cup mashed very ripe banana (about 1 medium banana)
⅓ cup maple syrup
½ cup vegetable oil
¼ cup whole milk plain Greek yogurt
2 teaspoons pure vanilla extract
2 large eggs

SERVES 10

NUTRITION INFORMATION (1 SLICE):
Calories: 247 | Added sugar: 1½ teaspoons or 6g | Carbohydrates: 30g | Sodium: 199mg | Saturated fat: 5% of calories or 1g | Fiber: 2g | Protein: 4g

SUPER MOIST BANANA BREAD

OURS = 0 TEASPOONS
THEIRS = 2½ TEASPOONS

Ingredients

Nonstick cooking spray

10 ounces Medjool dates, pitted (about 12 dates)

⅓ cup chopped pecans or walnuts (optional)

2 cups hot water

¾ cup whole milk plain Greek yogurt

2 medium very ripe bananas, mashed (about 1 cup)

1 large egg plus 1 large egg yolk, beaten

1 tablespoon pure vanilla extract

1½ cups all-purpose flour

1½ teaspoons baking powder

1 teaspoon baking soda

1 teaspoon salt

1 teaspoon ground cinnamon

½ teaspoon ground nutmeg

⅓ cup coconut oil or unsalted butter, at room temperature

SERVES 10

Ripe bananas, Medjool dates, and Greek yogurt give this banana bread its tender, moist crumb and delicious, natural sweetness with zero added sugar. Waiting for the bananas to fully ripen is critical to ensure that their natural sugars have time to develop, so don't rush this step. Your bananas should be dark and speckled. Toasted pecans add an extra layer of sweetness and texture.

1 Preheat the oven to 350°F. Line an 8½ × 4½-inch loaf pan with parchment paper, leaving 2 inches of overhang on each side, and coat with cooking spray.

2 Place the pitted dates in a medium bowl. Cover the dates with 2 cups hot water. Set aside until the dates are softened, about 10 minutes. Drain the dates, reserving 2 tablespoons of the soaking liquid.

3 If using, spread the pecans on a rimmed baking sheet and bake until lightly toasted, about 5 minutes. Set aside to cool.

4 Combine the dates, reserved soaking liquid, and yogurt in a food processor. Process until smooth and no flecks of date remain, about 2 minutes. Transfer the mixture to a medium bowl and add the mashed bananas, egg, egg yolk, and vanilla. Set aside.

5 Combine the flour, baking powder, baking soda, salt, cinnamon, nutmeg, and coconut oil in the bowl of a stand mixer fitted with a paddle attachment. Beat on low speed until the coconut oil and flour are a mealy powder, about 30 seconds. Add the date and banana mixture and continue beating until just combined and no visible flour remains.

6 Transfer the batter to the prepared pan, top with the nuts, if using, and bake until the bread is lightly browned and a toothpick inserted into the center comes out clean, 55 to 60 minutes. Let cool in the pan for 15 minutes, then use the parchment overhang to remove the bread from the pan. Cut into 10 slices and serve.

⭐ **MAKE AHEAD**
The banana bread will keep, tightly wrapped in plastic wrap, in the refrigerator for up to 3 days or in the freezer for up to 1 month.

NUTRITION INFORMATION (1 SLICE):
Calories: 264 | Added sugar: 0 teaspoons or 0g | Carbohydrates: 42g | Sodium: 314mg | Saturated fat: 24% of calories or 7g | Fiber: 3g | Protein: 5g

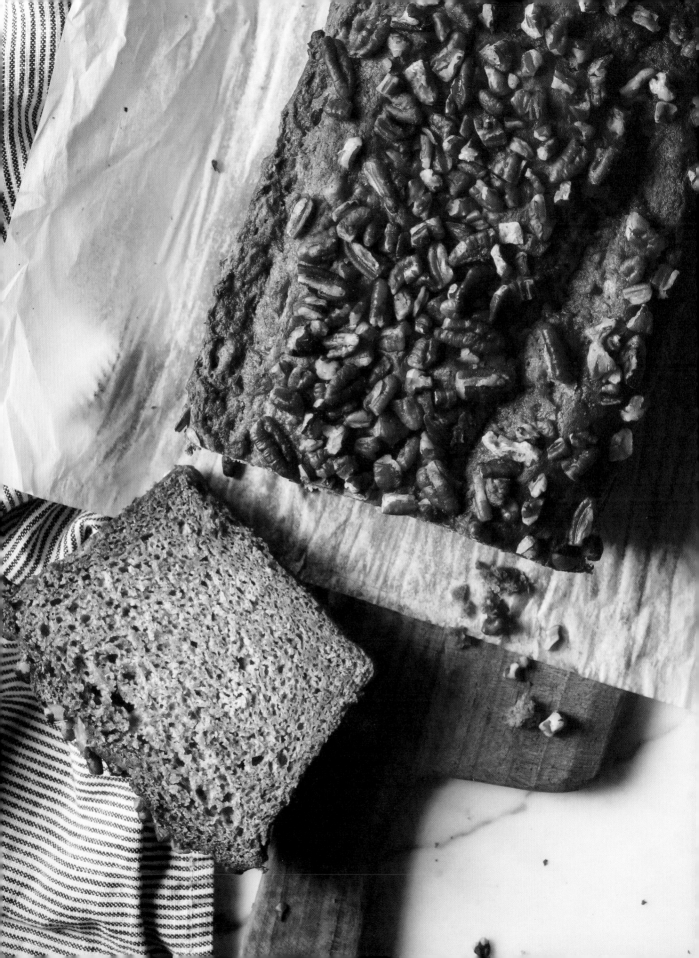

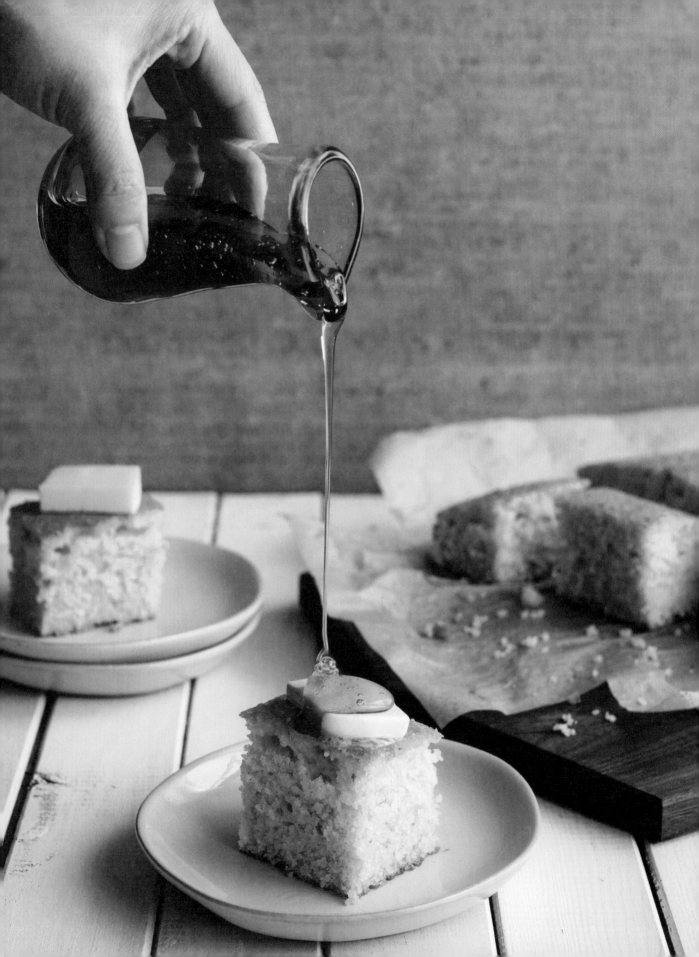

MAPLE–BROWN BUTTER CORN BREAD

OURS = ¾ TEASPOON
THEIRS = 1¾ TEASPOONS

Maple syrup adds sweetness and depth of flavor to this quick and easy corn bread. This recipe makes a big batch, so it's a wonderful complement to your summer cookouts. It pairs well with BBQ Chicken (page 96), Boston Baked Beans (page 97), and BBQ Chicken Chopped Salad (page 87), and is best served warm.

1 Preheat the oven to 425°F. Coat a 13 × 9-inch baking dish with cooking spray. Set aside.

2 Combine the melted butter and maple syrup in a medium bowl. Stir until well blended. Whisk in the buttermilk and eggs.

3 Whisk together the flour, cornmeal, baking powder, salt, and baking soda in a large bowl. Make a well in the center of the dry ingredients and pour in the butter mixture. Carefully incorporate the dry ingredients into the wet ingredients, being sure not to overmix. Stir until just combined.

4 Transfer the batter to the prepared dish and bake until golden brown and a toothpick inserted into the center comes out with a few moist crumbs, about 20 minutes. Let cool slightly, then cut into 30 pieces and serve warm or at room temperature, drizzled with a bit of maple syrup if you wish.

NOTE: The added sugar increases to just under 1 teaspoon if you drizzle your corn bread with maple syrup.

☆ **MAKE AHEAD**
The corn bread will keep, tightly wrapped in plastic wrap, at room temperature for up to 2 days.

Ingredients

Nonstick cooking spray
¾ cup (1½ sticks) unsalted butter, melted
⅓ cup plus 2 tablespoons maple syrup, plus extra for drizzling (optional)
2 cups low-fat buttermilk
4 large eggs
2 cups all-purpose flour
2 cups medium-grind yellow cornmeal
1 tablespoon baking powder
1 tablespoon kosher salt
1 teaspoon baking soda

SERVES 30

NUTRITION INFORMATION (1 PIECE WITHOUT MAPLE SYRUP DRIZZLE):
Calories: 136 | Added sugar: ¾ teaspoon or 3g | Carbohydrates: 18g | Sodium: 276mg | Saturated fat: 22% of calories or 3g | Fiber: 1g | Protein: 4g

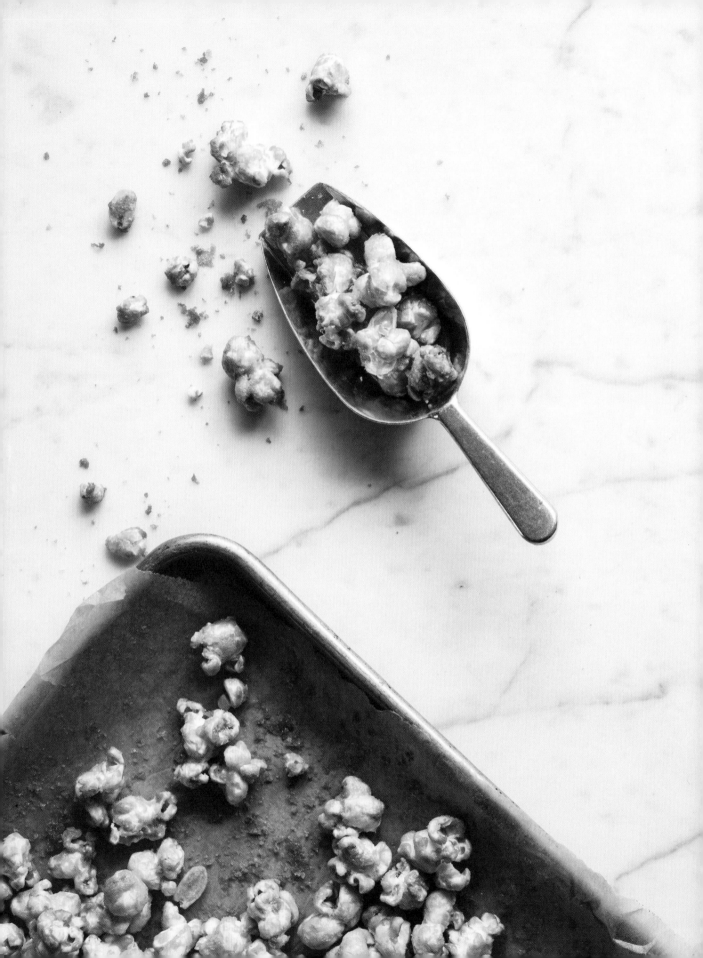

SNACKS

Snacks, especially the ones that typically show up in a lunch box, are often packed with a surprising amount of added sugar. Fruit-on-the-bottom yogurts, for example, can contain as much added sugar as a scoop of ice cream. We've taken your favorite nibbles and slashed the added sugar, so you can snack happy and healthy.

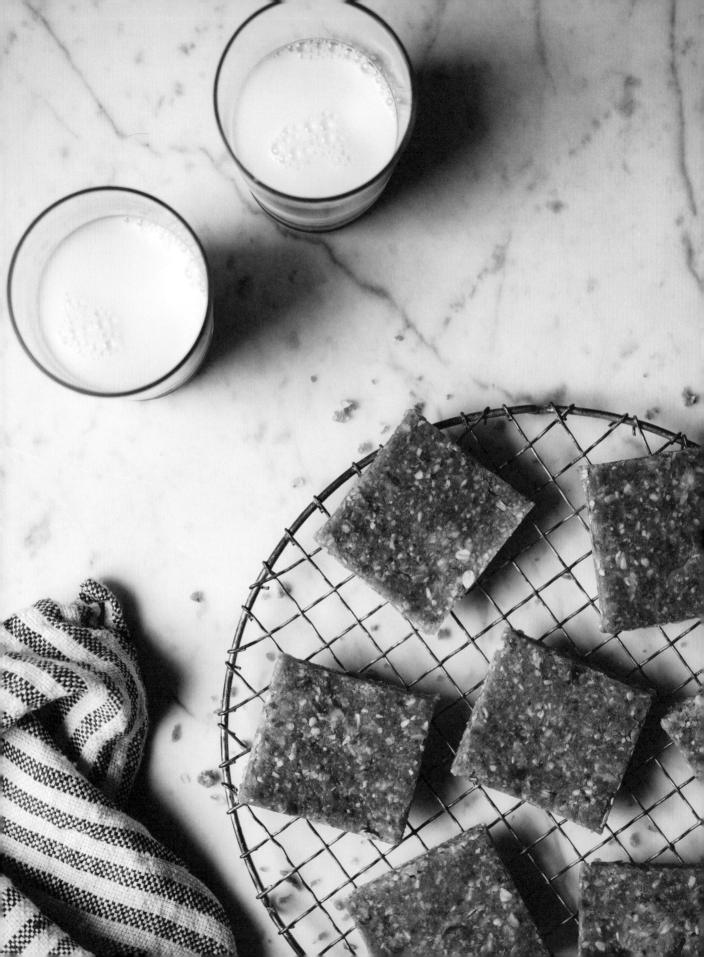

NO-BAKE PEANUT BUTTER ENERGY BARS

OURS = 0 TEASPOONS
THEIRS = 4¾ TEASPOONS

This no-bake energy bar is a riff on a popular brand's peanut butter bar, but with zero added sugar. Dates and peanut butter add natural sweetness, and tangerine juice adds just a touch of brightness and flavor, ensuring these bars satisfy the most intense snack cravings. They are filling! Because these bars aren't baked, they are a little softer than a packaged energy bar. For a firmer texture, serve straight from the refrigerator. If packing in a lunch box, include an ice pack to maintain the bars' texture.

Ingredients

1½ cups old-fashioned (rolled) oats

14 ounces Medjool dates, pitted (16 to 20 dates)

1 cup unsweetened peanut butter (creamy or chunky)

1 tablespoon ground flaxseed (optional)

2 teaspoons pure vanilla extract

½ teaspoon salt

2 tablespoons freshly squeezed tangerine juice (from 1 small tangerine)

MAKES 12 BARS

1 Line an 8 × 8-inch baking pan with parchment paper, leaving 2 inches of overhang on each side.

2 Place ½ cup of the oats in a food processor and pulse until a coarse flour forms, about 1 minute.

3 Add the remaining 1 cup oats, the dates, peanut butter, flaxseed, if using, vanilla, and salt to the processor and process until the dates are finely chopped, scraping the side of the bowl if necessary. Process until the mixture starts to clump together, 2 to 3 minutes.

4 Drizzle the juice into the mixture and pulse until incorporated.

5 Press the mixture into the baking pan, using an offset spatula to firmly press it down into an even layer. Refrigerate until firm, at least 30 minutes or overnight.

6 Cut into 12 bars, roughly 2 by 2½ inches each.

☺ **WHAT KIDS CAN DO**
Kids can squeeze the juice and press the mixture into the pan.

☆ **MAKE AHEAD**
The bars will keep, tightly wrapped in plastic wrap, in the refrigerator for up to 1 week or in the freezer for up to 1 month.

NUTRITION INFORMATION (1 BAR):
Calories: 266 | Added sugar: 0 teaspoons or 0g | Carbohydrates: 37g | Sodium: 98mg | Saturated fat: 6% of calories or 2g | Fiber: 5g | Protein: 7g

FRUIT-ON-THE-BOTTOM YOGURT PARFAITS

OURS = 1¾ TEASPOONS
THEIRS = 3½ TEASPOONS

Ingredients

10 ounces fresh
strawberries, hulled
and quartered
(about 1½ cups)

1½ tablespoons honey

½ teaspoon pure vanilla
extract

3 cups whole milk plain
yogurt or Greek yogurt

¼ cup chopped almonds or
Fruit and Nut Granola
(page 22; optional)

SERVES 4

These yogurt parfaits are a great alternative to packaged fruit-on-the-bottom yogurts, which can contain as much sugar as dessert. Naturally sweet fruit, a touch of honey, and vanilla add loads of flavor to these parfaits without loading up on added sugar. They're easy to prepare, making them great for after-school or lunch box snacks, or even a quick breakfast.

1 Set out 4 small glass jars or resealable glass containers.

2 Place the berries and 1 tablespoon of the honey in a small saucepan. Bring to a simmer over medium-high heat. Cook, gently mashing, until the fruit is tender and syrupy, about 5 minutes. Transfer to a medium bowl, stir in the vanilla, and let cool completely. You should have about ¾ cup of compote.

3 While the fruit is cooling, mix together the yogurt and the remaining ½ tablespoon of honey.

4 Spoon 3 tablespoons of the fruit compote into the bottom of each jar or container. Top with the yogurt mixture, evenly divided among the jars (about ¾ cup per jar). Top with nuts, if using, and serve immediately. If packing in a lunch box, use an airtight container and be sure to include an ice pack.

VARIATION: Use 10 ounces blueberries and/or peeled and sliced peaches instead of the strawberries.

☺ WHAT KIDS CAN DO
Kids can assemble the parfaits.

☆ MAKE AHEAD
The parfaits will keep in an airtight container in the refrigerator for up to 1 week.

NUTRITION INFORMATION (1 PARFAIT WITH WHOLE MILK PLAIN YOGURT, WITHOUT NUTS OR GRANOLA):
Calories: 160 | Added sugar: 1¾ teaspoons or 7g | Carbohydrates: 21g | Sodium: 86mg | Saturated fat: 23% of calories or 4g | Fiber: 1g | Protein: 7g

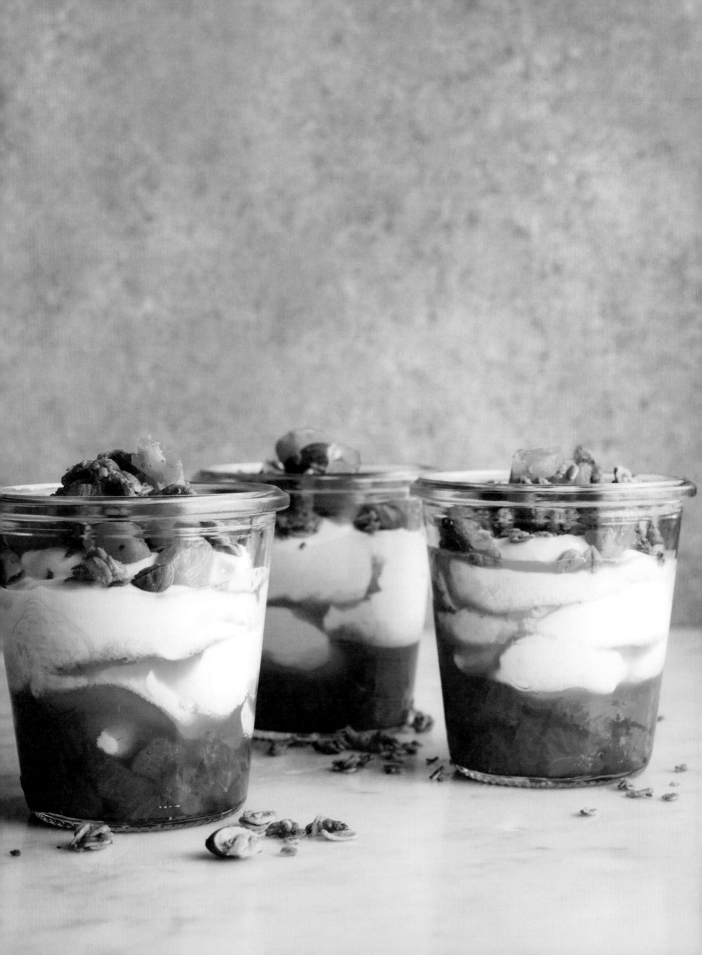

BAKED BBQ POTATO CHIPS

 OURS = 0 TEASPOONS*
THEIRS = ¼ TEASPOON

Ingredients

2¼ teaspoons sweet
    paprika
½ teaspoon salt
½ teaspoon smoked
    paprika
½ teaspoon tomato
    powder (see Note)
½ teaspoon packed light
    brown sugar
¼ teaspoon onion powder
⅛ teaspoon garlic powder
⅛ teaspoon freshly ground
    black pepper
1 pound Yukon Gold
    potatoes, peeled and
    sliced ⅛ inch thick on
    a mandoline
3 tablespoons extra-virgin
    olive oil

SERVES 8

These barbecue potato chips have plenty of smoky flavor with less sugar than conventional bagged chips. Because they are cut slightly thicker and baked rather than fried, these chips are best served the day they are made. You will see brown sugar listed in the ingredients, but it is a negligible amount; each serving of these chips has so little sugar that we consider them added sugar–free.

1 Preheat the oven to 375°F and set the oven racks in the upper and lower thirds of the oven. Line two rimmed baking sheets with parchment paper.

2 Make the BBQ seasoning: Whisk together the sweet paprika, salt, smoked paprika, tomato powder, brown sugar, onion powder, garlic powder, and pepper in a small bowl until combined. Set aside.

3 Place the potato slices in a large bowl. Using paper towels, blot away the excess moisture. Drizzle the potatoes with the oil. Using your hands, separate the potato slices and make sure each slice is coated in the oil.

4 Arrange the potato slices in a single layer on the prepared baking sheets. Wipe out the bowl and reserve it for later. Bake until the chips are crisp and golden with some brown areas, 30 to 33 minutes, rotating the baking sheets from top to bottom and 180 degrees halfway through baking.

5 Transfer the chips to the reserved bowl and sprinkle with the BBQ seasoning. Toss until the chips are evenly seasoned. Transfer the chips to a wire rack and let cool for 5 minutes. Serve immediately.

NOTE: Tomato powder can be purchased online. If you can't find it, increase the sweet paprika to 2½ teaspoons and the smoked paprika to ¾ teaspoon.

☺ **WHAT KIDS CAN DO**
Kids can arrange the potato slices on the pans and toss the baked chips in the BBQ seasoning.

NUTRITION INFORMATION (ABOUT 1½ OUNCES):
Calories: 93 | Added sugar: 0 teaspoons or 0g | Carbohydrates: 11g | Sodium: 150 mg | Saturated fat: 6% of calories or <1g | Fiber: 2g | Protein: 1g

*Negligible

MAPLE-ROASTED ALMONDS

 OURS: ¼ TEASPOON
THEIRS: 1 TEASPOON

Maple syrup and cinnamon add just the right amount of sweetness to these roasted almonds. Perfect for your snack table at the big game, or for munching at movie night, these little sweeties satisfy snack cravings in the healthiest of ways.

1 Preheat the oven to 325°F. Line a rimmed baking sheet with parchment paper.

2 In a medium bowl, whisk together the maple syrup, salt, and cinnamon. Add the almonds and stir well to evenly coat the nuts with the maple mixture.

3 Spread the almonds on the prepared baking sheet in a single layer and bake until toasty, 12 to 15 minutes.

4 Remove from the oven and let cool completely. Once cool, break apart any almonds sticking together. These almonds are best served right off the pan.

Ingredients

1½ tablespoons maple syrup
1 teaspoon salt
1 teaspoon ground cinnamon
3 cups raw, unsalted almonds

MAKES 3 CUPS

NUTRITION INFORMATION (¼ CUP):
Calories: 216 | Added sugar: ¼ teaspoon or 1g | Carbohydrates: 10g | Sodium: 194mg | Saturated fat: 6% of calories or 1g | Fiber: 5g | Protein: 8g

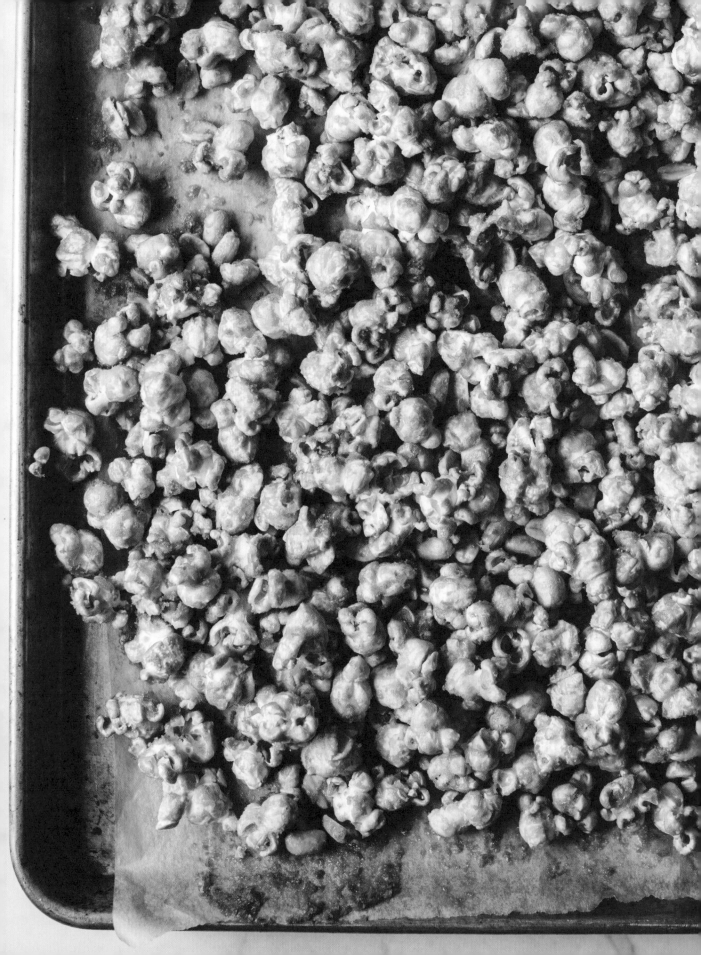

MAPLE CARAMEL CORN

OURS = 1¼ TEASPOONS
THEIRS = 3¼ TEASPOONS

Maple syrup adds delicious flavor to this low-sugar snack that's reminiscent of the classic caramel corn in the box. Baking soda is the secret. It helps to create a light and crispy texture that is irresistible. You will need to work quickly before the caramel hardens, so make sure you have everything ready to go and measured before you start making the caramel.

1 Preheat the oven to 250°F and line a rimmed baking sheet with parchment paper.

2 Place the popcorn in a large bowl and add the peanuts, if using.

3 Melt the butter in a small saucepan over medium-high heat. Add the maple syrup and salt. Bring to a boil and continue to boil for a full 5 minutes, stirring often, until the mixture flows in a steady stream from the spoon. You can tell it's ready if you place a few drops on a cool plate and you can see the mixture start to thicken as it cools, or when it reaches 230°F on a digital or candy thermometer. Be careful! The caramel is very hot.

4 Remove the caramel from the heat and carefully stir in the vanilla and baking soda. The mixture will foam up.

5 Quickly pour the caramel over the popcorn and peanuts and toss with a spatula until coated.

6 While the mixture is still hot, spread it in the pan in an even layer. Bake until the popcorn is light and crispy, about 45 minutes, stirring every 15 minutes.

7 Cool briefly, then serve.

NOTE: Prepare the popcorn in oil or an air popper according to the package directions.

⚡ **QUICK TIP**
You can also use microwave popcorn. You'll need about 1½ bags, depending on the yield. Use the kind with no added salt or butter.

☆ **MAKE AHEAD**
The caramel corn tastes best the day it is made but will keep in an airtight container at room temperature for 2 to 3 days.

Ingredients

11 cups freshly popped popcorn (from about ⅓ cup popcorn kernels; see Note)

½ cup roasted salted peanuts (optional)

4 tablespoons (½ stick) unsalted butter

½ cup plus 2 tablespoons pure maple syrup

¼ teaspoon salt

1 teaspoon pure vanilla extract

½ teaspoon baking soda

MAKES 11 CUPS

NUTRITION INFORMATION (½ CUP WITHOUT PEANUTS):
Calories: 64 | Added sugar: 1¼ teaspoons or 5g | Carbohydrates: 8g | Sodium: 56mg | Saturated fat: 21% of calories or 2g | Fiber: <1g | Protein: <1g

CHOCOLATE-DRIZZLED GRAHAM CRACKERS

OURS: ½ TEASPOON
THEIRS: 1¼ TEASPOONS

Ingredients

1½ cups all-purpose flour

¾ cup whole-wheat flour

⅓ cup sugar

2 teaspoons ground
cinnamon

1 teaspoon baking powder

1 teaspoon salt

½ teaspoon baking soda

½ cup (1 stick) cold
unsalted butter,
cubed

1 tablespoon pure
vanilla extract

1 ounce dark chocolate
chips (about 3
tablespoons)

1½ teaspoons coconut oil
or canola oil

MAKES 18 LARGE SQUARE CRACKERS

☺ **WHAT KIDS CAN DO**
Kids can prick the
crackers and drizzle
on the chocolate.

☆ **MAKE AHEAD**
The crackers will
keep stored in an
airtight container
in the refrigerator
for up to 3 days.

Because graham flour can be tough to find, this recipe uses a combination of whole-wheat and all-purpose flours—the combo creates that classic graham cracker depth of flavor without compromising flakiness. Granulated sugar works best here to achieve the perfect level of sweetness with less than half the added sugar you'd typically find in packaged chocolate-covered grahams.

1 Combine the flours, sugar, cinnamon, baking powder, salt, and baking soda in a food processor. Pulse until combined, about 10 seconds. Add the butter and process until the mixture resembles coarse cornmeal, about 15 seconds. Add ¼ cup water and the vanilla and process until the dough comes together, about 30 seconds. Transfer to a large bowl and knead a few times. The dough should be slightly sticky and soft, but not wet. Cover with plastic wrap and let rest at room temperature for 30 minutes.

2 Preheat the oven to 300°F.

3 Divide the dough into two equal pieces and shape each into a square about 1 inch thick. Working with one piece at a time, roll between two large sheets of parchment paper into a rectangle about ⅛ inch thick (about 16 inches long and 8 inches wide). Remove the top piece of parchment and score the surface of the dough into eighteen 2½-inch squares. Then score each square down the center to create 36 rectangles. Prick each rectangle multiple times with a fork. Transfer the parchment with the dough to a rimmed baking sheet and bake until the crackers are golden around the edges and firm, about 30 minutes. Let cool completely. Break apart on scored lines into squares or rectangles.

4 Meanwhile, in a bowl set over a pot of simmering water, melt together the chocolate and coconut oil. Let cool slightly. Drizzle the chocolate over the crackers and refrigerate until the chocolate is hardened, 10 minutes.

NUTRITION INFORMATION (1 LARGE SQUARE CRACKER):
Calories: 65 | Added sugar: ½ teaspoon or 2g | Carbohydrates: 8g | Sodium: 83mg | Saturated fat: 25% of calories or 2g | Fiber: 2g | Protein: 4g

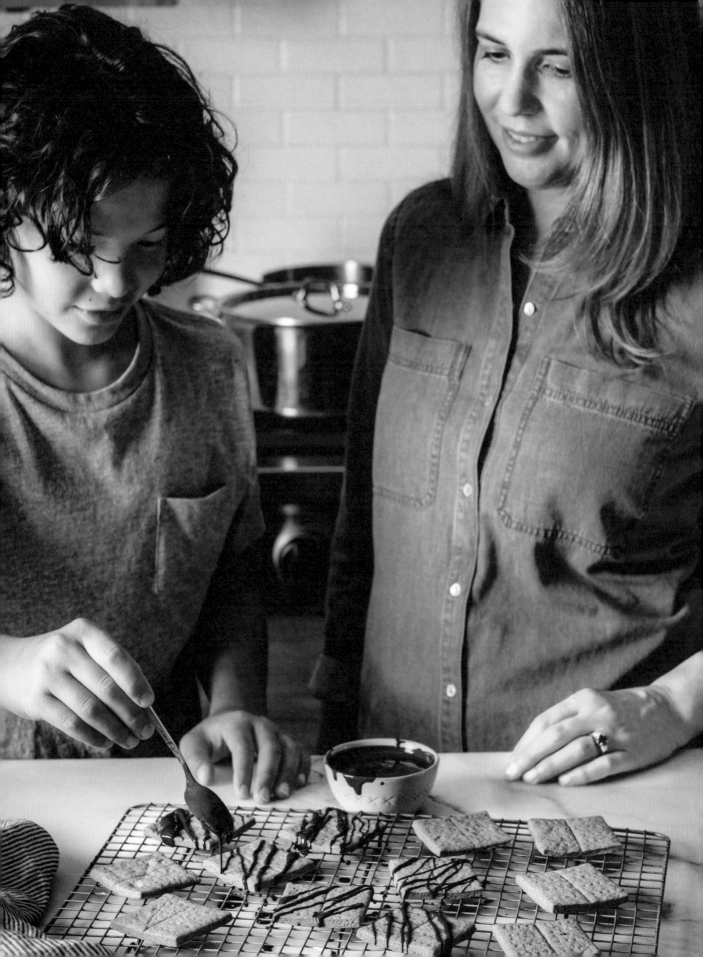

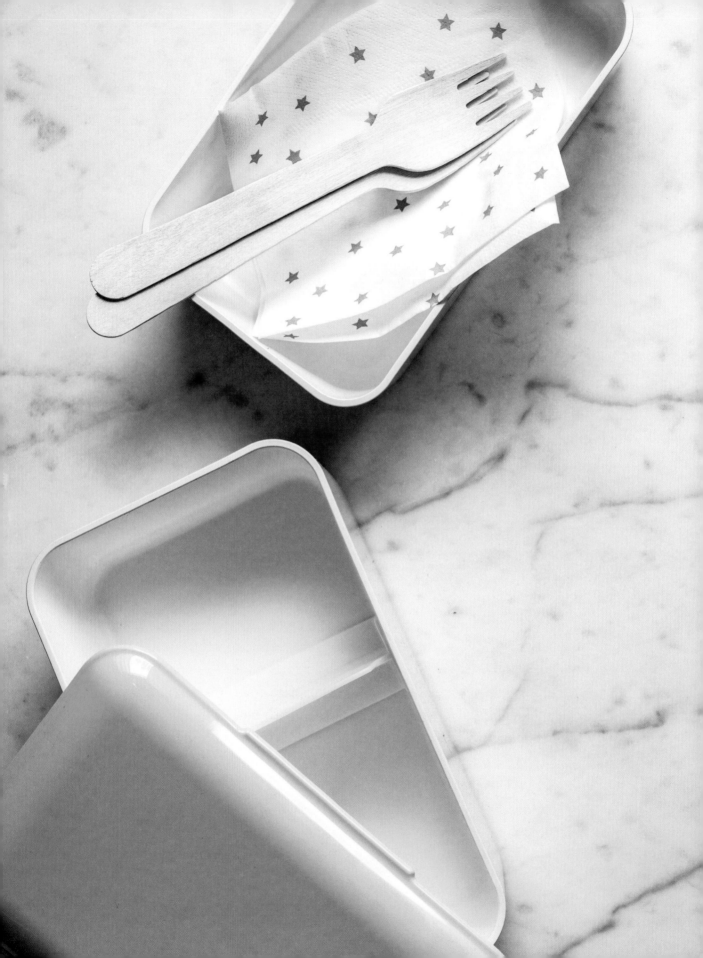

LUNCHES AND SALADS

Packing a healthy lunch that your kids will actually eat can be a challenge. Added sugar (and sodium) looms large in prepackaged kids' lunches, so we've pulled together delicious lunch box meals that are easy to make *and* low in sugar and sodium. The main source of added sugar in lunches is usually sweet spreads and sauces. We've remastered our favorites and worked them into quick and easy packable meals. To save time and make weekday mornings less stressful, it's best to make the spreads and sauces in advance if you can.

We've also taken the most beloved hearty restaurant salads—like tangy Chinese chicken salad and a popular pizza chain's famous BBQ chicken chopped salad—and reworked them with new dressings that maximize flavor with low added sugar or none at all. Making your own salad dressings at home is easy and results in salads with much more flavor and considerably less added sugar.

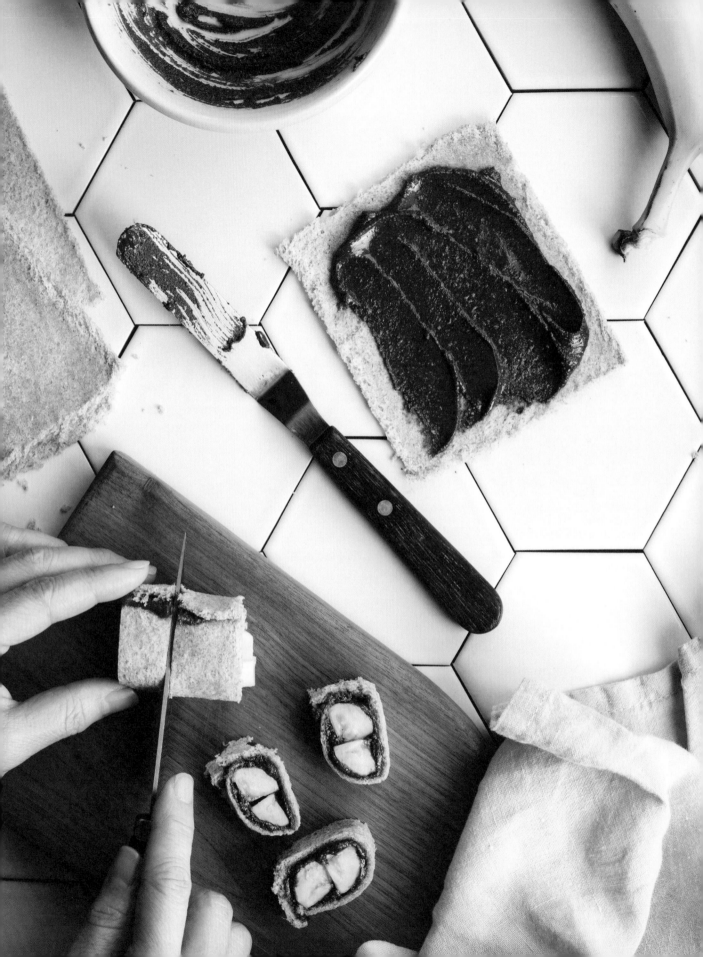

NEWTELLA AND BANANA ROLL UPS

OURS = 1 TEASPOON
THEIRS = 5¼ TEASPOONS

These adorable chocolate and banana roll ups are a great addition to any lunch box. They are super quick to make, pack easily, and satisfy your little ones with a delicious and healthy school lunch. Since many kids have nut allergies or go to a school that is nut free, use Nut-Free Newtella for these sandwich bites. The combination of chocolate, pumpkin and sunflower seeds, and bananas is irresistible. Feel free to use hazelnut-based Newtella if you prefer.

Ingredients

4 slices whole-wheat
sandwich bread
1 medium banana
¼ cup Nut-Free Newtella
(page 197) or Newtella
(page 196)

SERVES 2

1 Roll each slice of bread with a rolling pin until flattened to about 1⁄16-inch thickness. Trim the crusts from the bread.

2 Peel the banana and trim the ends until the banana is the same length as the bread. Quarter the banana lengthwise, then cut each quarter in half lengthwise to yield 8 long strips.

3 To assemble the roll ups, spread 1 tablespoon of the newtella evenly on a slice of bread. Place 2 banana strips along the bottom edge of the bread. Gently roll the bread away from you, folding the bread over the fruit and pressing the seam to seal the roll. Repeat with the remaining bread, spread, and fruit.

4 Cut each roll crosswise into 6 equal pieces. Place the roll ups cut side up in a lunch box. They are best eaten the day they are made.

☺ **WHAT KIDS CAN DO**
Kids can roll out the bread and spread the newtella.

NUTRITION INFORMATION (12 PIECES WITH NUT-FREE NEWTELLA):
Calories: 373 | Added sugar: 1 teaspoon or 4g | Carbohydrates: 45g | Sodium: 365mg | Saturated fat: 9% of calories or 4g | Fiber: 8g | Protein: 14g

STRAWBERRY AND CREAM CHEESE SAMMY

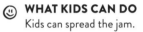 OURS: 1 TEASPOON
THEIRS = 5½ TEASPOONS

Ingredients

2 tablespoons Three-Ingredient Strawberry Jam (page 198)
2 slices whole-wheat sandwich bread
1 tablespoon cream cheese, at room temperature

MAKES 1 SANDWICH

This sweet and creamy sandwich is a great alternative to PB&J for breakfast or lunch. The simple homemade strawberry jam contributes natural sweetness without loads of added sugar. To quickly soften the cream cheese, place it in a microwave-safe bowl and microwave on high for 8 to 10 seconds.

1 Spread the jam evenly on one slice of the bread. Spread the cream cheese evenly on the other slice of bread.

2 Stack the two slices of bread together so that the jam and cream cheese fillings are both in the center.

3 Cut the sandwich in half. Wrap each half tightly in plastic wrap or place in a lidded sandwich container. Place in a lunch box along with an ice pack.

☺ **WHAT KIDS CAN DO**
Kids can spread the jam.

☆ **MAKE AHEAD**
This sandwich can be made the night before and stored, tightly wrapped in plastic wrap, in the refrigerator.

NUTRITION INFORMATION (1 SANDWICH):
Calories: 215 | Added sugar: 1 teaspoon or 4g | Carbohydrates: 30g | Sodium: 311mg | Saturated fat: 14% of calories or 3g | Fiber: 5g | Protein: 8g

TURKEY PANINI
WITH CRANBERRY SAUCE

 OURS: ¾ TEASPOON
THEIRS: 3 TEASPOONS

This satisfying, cheesy griddled sandwich is loaded with some of your Thanksgiving favorites, such as roast turkey, cranberry sauce, spinach, and red onion. It's best when eaten piping hot, but it is also great served cold, packed up in a lunch box. It's an excellent way to use up leftover Thanksgiving fixings.

1 Brush one side of each slice of bread with the olive oil. Flip the bread oiled side down. Spread the mayonnaise on one slice of bread, spread the cranberry sauce on the other slice of bread.

2 Place the cheese on top of the mayonnaise-covered bread slice, followed by the turkey, spinach, and onion. Cover with the other piece of bread, cranberry-sauce side down.

3 Warm a large nonstick skillet over medium-high heat until hot. Place the sandwich in the skillet and set another heavy skillet or pan on top. Push down on the inside of the second pan to compress the sandwich as it cooks, using an oven mitt or kitchen towel to protect your hand. Cook until the bottom of the sandwich is golden brown and crispy, 45 to 60 seconds.

4 Remove the second pan and use a large spatula to flip the sandwich over. Replace the second pan on top of the sandwich and continue cooking in the same manner until the other side of the sandwich is golden brown and the cheese is melted, 30 to 60 seconds.

5 Transfer the panini to a cutting board and cut in half with a sharp knife. Serve immediately, or to pack in a lunch box, let cool on a wire rack for 10 minutes before wrapping each half in aluminum foil.

⚡ **QUICK TIP**
Use low-sodium or no-sodium-added sliced deli turkey instead of homemade roasted turkey. If using low-sodium deli turkey, this will increase the sodium content per serving by 90 to 115 milligrams depending on the brand you choose.

Ingredients

- 2 slices whole-wheat sandwich bread
- 1 teaspoon extra-virgin olive oil
- 1½ teaspoons mayonnaise
- 2 tablespoons Cranberry Sauce (page 191)
- 1 slice provolone cheese (1 ounce)
- 2 ounces thinly sliced roasted turkey breast, preferably homemade (see sidebar below)
- ¼ cup lightly packed baby spinach
- 2 thin slices red onion

MAKES 1 SANDWICH

To roast turkey breast from scratch, season a 2-pound bone-in, skin-on turkey breast half lightly with salt and place on an aluminum foil–lined, rimmed baking sheet. Roast in a 400°F oven until a thermometer inserted into the thickest part of the breast, away from the bone, registers 160°F. Let rest for 10 minutes before peeling away the skin and slicing. Or let cool before wrapping the turkey tightly in plastic wrap and refrigerating for up to 1 week. The turkey will be easier to slice thinly when it is completely cold.

NUTRITION INFORMATION (1 SANDWICH):
Calories: 455 | Added sugar: ¾ teaspoon or 3g | Carbohydrates: 37g | Sodium: 673 mg | Saturated fat: 14% of calories or 7g | Fiber: 6g | Protein: 30g

SALMON YAKI ONIGIRI
(GRILLED RICE BALLS)

OURS: ¼ TEASPOON
THEIRS: 1¼ TEASPOON

Ingredients

1¼ cups short-grain
  white rice
½ teaspoon salt
1 tablespoon vegetable oil
1 fillet (4 ounces) skin-on
  salmon, preferably
  wild-caught, about
  1 inch thick
3 tablespoons Pineapple
  Teriyaki Glaze
  (page 186)

SERVES 4

Yaki onigiri is made from white rice that is formed into a compact triangular shape, grilled until crisp and lightly browned, and brushed with a salty-sweet soy glaze. This handheld Japanese treat can be prepared plain or with a small amount of filling. Here, we've included cooked salmon and used our Pineapple Teriyaki Glaze to sweeten the outside. While yaki onigiri is best served hot for maximum crispness, it is no less delicious tucked into a lunch box (with an ice pack) and eaten several hours later, although it will be softer and chewier in texture.

1 Place the rice in a fine-mesh strainer and rinse under cold water until the water runs clear. Transfer the rice to a small saucepan and add 1½ cups water and ¼ teaspoon plus ⅛ teaspoon of the salt. Bring to a boil over medium-high heat, stir the rice, then reduce the heat to low.

2 Cover and cook until the rice is tender and the liquid is absorbed, about 15 minutes. Remove from the heat and let stand, covered, for 10 minutes. Fluff the rice with a fork. Set aside, uncovered, and let cool slightly. You should have about 4 cups of rice.

3 Meanwhile, in a small nonstick skillet, heat 1 teaspoon of the oil over medium-high heat. Sprinkle the salmon on all sides with the remaining ⅛ teaspoon salt. Add the salmon to the skillet and cook, turning occasionally with a spatula, until golden brown on all sides and the flesh flakes apart easily when tested with the tip of a paring knife, about 8 minutes total. Transfer to a small bowl and let cool for 10 minutes. Remove and discard the skin, then flake the fish finely with a fork. You should have ½ cup salmon.

Recipe continues

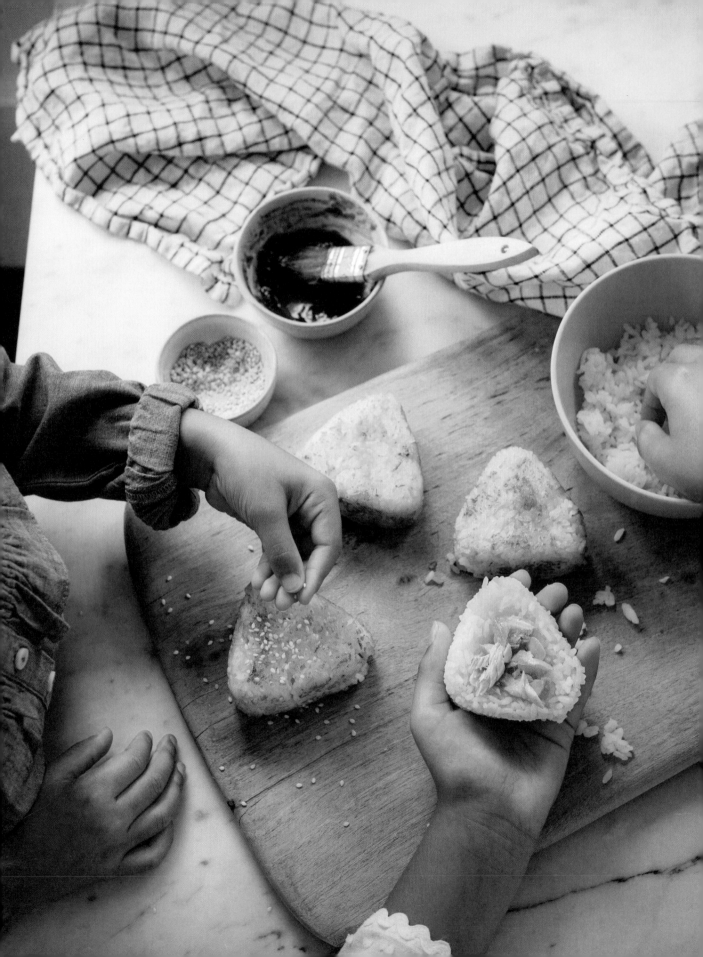

4 When the rice is still warm but cool enough to handle, form the onigiri: Lightly wet your hands. For each onigiri, scoop out ½ cup lightly packed rice. Take about two thirds of this rice and place it in the palm of your nondominant hand. Using the fingertips of your other hand, gently press a shallow well into the center of the rice and fill it with 1 tablespoon of the flaked salmon. Add the remaining one third of the rice on top. Use both hands to gently press and shape the rice into a triangular form. Set the onigiri aside on a plastic wrap–lined plate and repeat with the remaining rice and salmon.

5 If making ahead, wrap each onigiri individually with plastic wrap. Refrigerate up to overnight and unwrap just before pan-frying.

6 Brush the remaining 2 teaspoons oil evenly on a large nonstick or cast-iron skillet and warm over medium heat. Arrange the rice balls in a single layer and cook until lightly browned and crispy on the bottom. Flip with a spatula and cook until the other side is lightly browned and crispy, 5 to 7 minutes total.

7 Using a pastry brush, brush the top and sides of the onigiri with the teriyaki glaze. Gently turn the onigiri over and cook until lightly browned on the bottom, about 30 seconds. Meanwhile, brush the other side with the remaining glaze. Turn the onigiri over and cook until lightly browned on the other side, about 30 seconds.

8 Using a spatula, transfer the onigiri to a platter. Serve immediately, or let cool slightly and wrap individually with plastic wrap, pack in a lunch box with an ice pack, and eat within 4 to 5 hours.

⚡ **QUICK TIP**
To save time, you can use ½ cup drained, flaked boneless, skinless canned pink salmon from a 5- to 6-ounce can. The amount of sodium will be slightly more or less than the original recipe, depending on the brand used.

☺ **WHAT KIDS CAN DO**
Kids can help mold the rice balls.

NUTRITION INFORMATION (2 BALLS):
Calories: 327 | Added sugar: ¼ teaspoon or 1g | Carbohydrates: 56g | Sodium: 470mg | Saturated fat: 2% of calories or 1g | Fiber: 0g | Protein: 10g

COLD SESAME NOODLES
WITH TOFU AND VEGETABLES

OURS = 1¼ TEASPOONS
THEIRS = 3 TO 4 TEASPOONS

This tamed version of spicy Chinese noodles is wonderful for kids, especially if you use just 1 teaspoon of chile oil to start. This recipe is a great option for packaged lunches, but you can also serve it as a DIY dinner. Place the sauce in a pitcher and all the noodle ingredients in separate bowls, then have everyone assemble their noodle bowls and drizzle with sauce to taste. Feel free to mix it up with extra or different toppings, such as broccoli slaw, leftover cooked and shredded chicken, or sautéed shrimp.

1 Make the sauce: Whisk together the soy sauce, vinegar, sugar, sesame oil, and chile oil in a medium bowl until the sugar is dissolved. Stir in the garlic and ginger.

2 Make the noodles: Bring a pot of unsalted water to boil for the noodles and have a strainer ready in the sink. Cook the noodles according to the package directions, then strain and rinse with cold running water, gently tossing the noodles, until cooled all the way through. Shake to drain well.

3 Place the noodles in a large bowl with the tofu, cucumber, carrots, and all but a small amount of the green onions, cilantro, and peanuts. Add the sauce and toss to coat. If needed, drizzle in more sesame oil. Divide among

four bowls or containers and top with the remaining green onions, cilantro, and peanuts and the sesame seeds. Serve extra chile oil on the side, if you like. If packing in a lunch box, use a resealable container and an ice pack.

NOTE: We use unseasoned baked tofu for this. If using teriyaki-flavored baked tofu, your added sugar total for this recipe will increase to 2 teaspoons per serving.

😊 **WHAT KIDS CAN DO**
Kids can make the sauce, tasting as they go to get the right level of spiciness.

☆ **MAKE AHEAD**
The sauce will keep in an airtight container in the refrigerator for up to 2 weeks. The noodles don't keep well.

Ingredients

- 3 tablespoons low-sodium soy sauce
- 2 tablespoons white vinegar
- 1½ tablespoons sugar
- 1 tablespoon toasted (dark) sesame oil, plus more as needed
- 1 to 2 teaspoons chile oil or sriracha, plus more for serving
- 1 teaspoon chopped garlic
- 1 teaspoon peeled and grated fresh ginger
- 12 ounces dried Chinese-style thin wheat or egg noodles, or angel hair pasta
- 1 package (6 ounces) baked tofu, cut into matchsticks (see Note)
- ½ cup cucumber matchsticks
- ½ cup carrot matchsticks
- ¼ cup minced green onions
- ¼ cup fresh cilantro leaves
- ¼ cup unsalted roasted peanuts, roughly chopped
- 2 tablespoons toasted sesame seeds

SERVES 4

NUTRITION INFORMATION (1 SERVING WITH UNSEASONED TOFU):
Calories: 500 | Added sugar: 1¼ teaspoons or 5g | Carbohydrates: 76g | Sodium: 455mg | Saturated fat: 4% of calories or 2g | Fiber: 6g | Protein: 19g

CHINESE BBQ PORK FRIED RICE ⊗

OURS = 0 TEASPOONS*
THEIRS = 5 TEASPOONS

Ingredients

2 tablespoons vegetable oil

4 cups cooked white rice, at room temperature

2 teaspoons minced garlic

2 medium carrots (about 6 ounces), peeled and chopped into small dice

1 small onion, peeled and diced (about ½ cup)

6 ounces Sweet and Sticky Chinese BBQ Pork Roast (page 108), chopped into medium dice

1 cup frozen green peas

2 large eggs

2 teaspoons low-sodium soy sauce

SERVES 4

⚡ **QUICK TIP**
Toss 6 ounces chopped rotisserie chicken, skin removed, with 1 tablespoon Chinese Hoisin Sauce (page 187) to substitute for the pork.

☆ **MAKE AHEAD**
The fried rice will keep in an airtight container in the refrigerator for up to 2 days.

Fried rice is a lunch-box saver. It's easily packed in a thermos, and you can incorporate a variety of different vegetables, depending on what you need to use up in your fridge. Sweet and Sticky Chinese BBQ Pork Roast is the star here. The secret to restaurant-quality fried rice is to dry out the rice, so it's best to make a batch of rice ahead of time and let it fully cool on your counter before preparing this dish. Freshly cooked rice will have too much moisture, causing the fried rice to stick together.

1 Heat a large wok or large skillet over high heat. Add 1 tablespoon of the oil, swirl to coat the pan, then add the rice. Using a large spatula, spread the rice evenly in the pan, breaking up any large clumps. Let the rice cook, untouched, until the bottom is crisp, 2 minutes. Toss gently in the pan, scraping up any crispy bits, and cook until the rice is warmed through, about 1 minute more.

2 Make a well in the middle of the pan. Add 1½ teaspoons of the oil to the well, then add the garlic, carrots, and onion. Cook until the vegetables soften and begin to brown on the edges,

about 2 minutes. Add the pork and peas and stir until the peas are thawed (you may need to break up additional clumps of rice), about 1 minute more.

3 Make another well in the middle of the pan. Add the remaining 1½ teaspoons of oil to the well, let it heat momentarily, then add the eggs. Scramble the eggs until they are cooked through, about 1 minute, then mix with the rice to combine.

4 Add the soy sauce and toss to coat. Serve immediately. If packing in a lunch box, use a preheated thermos to ensure that the rice stays warm.

NUTRITION INFORMATION (1 SERVING):
Calories: 469 | Added sugar: 0 teaspoons or 0g | Carbohydrates: 57g | Sodium: 480mg | Saturated fat: 8% of calories or 4g | Fiber: 4g | Protein: 19g

*Negligible

ALPHABET SOUP

OURS = 0 TEASPOONS
THEIRS = 2¼ TEASPOONS

Grated sweet potato gives this chock-full-of-vegetables, tomato-based soup plenty of body and sweetness. Feel free to substitute vegetable broth for the chicken broth if you'd like to make it vegetarian. If you can't find alphabet pasta, use small shells or ditalini instead.

1 Heat the oil in a Dutch oven over medium heat. Add the onion and cook until softened and translucent, about 8 minutes, stirring occasionally. Add the carrots, celery, potato, and sweet potato and sauté for 5 minutes more.

2 Add the garlic and cook until fragrant, about 30 seconds. Stir in the broth, tomato puree, Italian seasoning, salt, and pepper. Bring to a boil over medium-high heat.

3 Reduce the heat to medium-low, cover, and cook until the potato

and carrots are nearly tender, about 10 minutes. Stir in the pasta, cover, and cook for 7 minutes.

4 Stir in the peas and corn, cover, and cook until the pasta and vegetables are tender, about 5 minutes more. Serve immediately. If packing in a lunch box, use a thermos.

☆ **MAKE AHEAD**
If you'd like to make this ahead, cook the pasta separately from the rest of the soup according to the package directions. Store it in an airtight container in the refrigerator until ready to use.

NUTRITION INFORMATION (1½ CUPS):
Calories: 226 | Added sugar: 0 teaspoons or 0g | Carbohydrates: 36g | Sodium: 385mg | Saturated fat: 5% of calories or 1g | Fiber: 5g | Protein: 10g

Ingredients

2 tablespoons extra-virgin olive oil

2 cups chopped sweet onion (about 1 large onion)

2 medium carrots, peeled and sliced into ¼-inch-thick coins

1 celery rib, halved lengthwise, then cut crosswise into ½-inch pieces

1 medium Yukon Gold potato (8 ounces), peeled and cut into ½-inch dice

1 small sweet potato (3½ to 4 ounces), peeled and grated on the large holes of a box grater

3 cloves garlic, peeled and minced

6 cups low-sodium chicken broth

1 cup tomato puree

1 teaspoon Italian seasoning

½ teaspoon salt

¼ teaspoon freshly ground black pepper

1 cup alphabet pasta

½ cup frozen green peas

½ cup frozen corn

SERVES 6

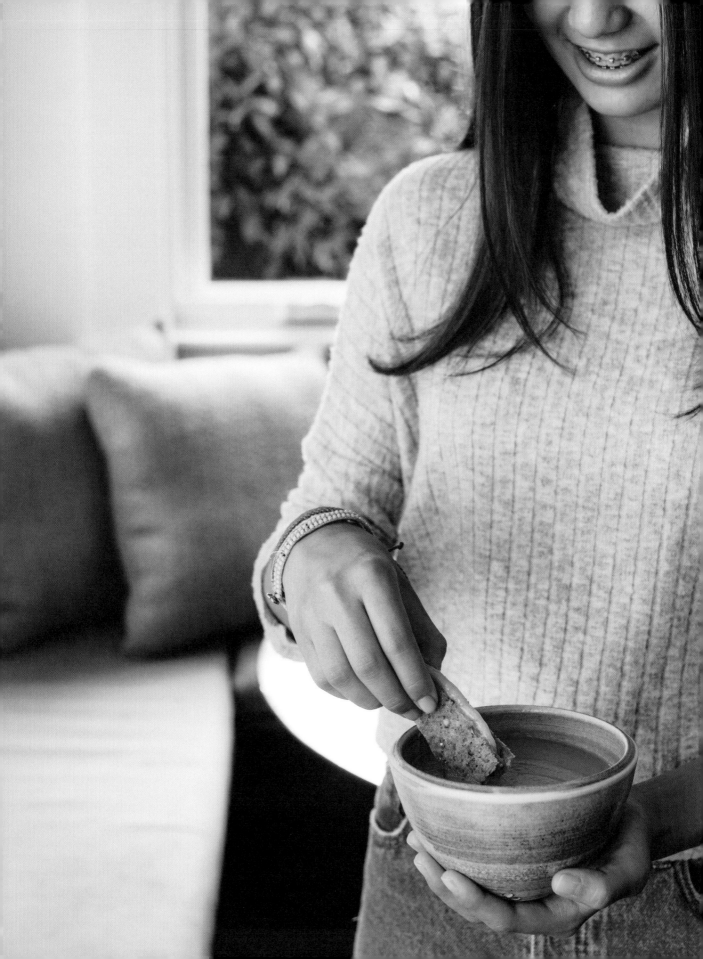

CREAMY TOMATO SOUP

OURS = 0 TEASPOONS
THEIRS = 1 TEASPOON

Unless made with perfectly ripe tomatoes, tomato soup can often taste acidic. That's why it's often tamed with the addition of sugar. Here, the boost of sweetness comes from carrots instead, which also thicken the soup and add a nice, velvety texture. Pair with grilled Cheddar cheese sandwiches cut into sticks for dipping.

Ingredients

- 2 tablespoons extra-virgin olive oil
- 2 cups chopped sweet onion (about 1 large onion)
- 8 ounces carrots (about 3 medium carrots), peeled and thinly sliced
- 3 cloves garlic, peeled and minced
- 2 cans (14.5 ounces each) no-salt-added diced tomatoes, with their juice
- ¾ teaspoon salt
- ¼ teaspoon freshly ground black pepper
- ¼ cup lightly packed fresh basil leaves

SERVES 7

1 Heat the oil in a large saucepan over medium heat. Add the onion and carrots. Cover and cook until very soft, about 10 minutes, uncovering the pot to stir occasionally.

2 Add the garlic and cook until fragrant, about 30 seconds. Stir in the tomatoes and 3¼ cups water, along with the salt and pepper. Bring to a boil over medium-high heat.

3 Reduce the heat to medium and simmer for 10 minutes. Remove the soup from the heat. Stir in the basil.

4 Working in two batches, carefully transfer the soup to a blender and blend until smooth and creamy. Return the soup to the pot, reheat if necessary. Ladle into individual bowls and serve. If packing in a lunch box, use a thermos.

⭐ **MAKE AHEAD**
The soup will keep in an airtight container in the refrigerator for up to 5 days or in the freezer for up to 2 months.

NUTRITION INFORMATION (1 CUP):
Calories: 89 | Added sugar: 0 teaspoons or 0g | Carbohydrates: 7g | Sodium: 290 mg | Saturated fat: 5% of calories or 1g | Fiber: 2g | Protein: 1g

FALL HARVEST MASON JAR SALAD
WITH CREAMY POPPY SEED DRESSING

Ingredients

½ cup farro

⅛ teaspoon plus a pinch
of salt

1 cup diced, peeled
butternut squash
(cut in ½-inch pieces)

1 teaspoon extra-virgin
olive oil

¼ cup Creamy Poppy
Seed Dressing
(page 194)

¼ cup pomegranate seeds

3 ounces lacinato kale,
ribs removed, leaves
very thinly sliced
(about 3½ loosely
packed cups)

4 ounces Brussels sprouts
(6 to 8 sprouts),
root ends trimmed,
very thinly sliced
(about 1¼ cups)

¼ cup roasted salted
pumpkin seeds

2 tablespoons shaved
Parmesan cheese

**SERVES 2 AS A MAIN DISH
OR 4 AS A SIDE SALAD**

Crispy, chewy, crunchy, and tender—this colorful autumnal salad has a variety of textures to keep things interesting. The combination of farro, pumpkin seeds, and Parmesan cheese provides plenty of savory flavor as well as protein—without meat. Creamy Poppy Seed Dressing brings it all together with less than half the sugar of a store-bought dressing. This salad can be easily doubled.

1 Preheat the oven to 400°F.

2 Place the farro in a strainer and rinse with cold water. Transfer the farro to a small saucepan with 1½ cups water and ⅛ teaspoon of the salt. Bring to a boil over medium-high heat, then reduce the heat to medium-low and simmer, partially covered, until tender, about 30 minutes. Return the farro to the strainer to drain any excess water. Spread the farro on a plate and let it cool completely.

3 Meanwhile, line a rimmed baking sheet with aluminum foil and place the butternut squash on top. Drizzle the squash with the oil and sprinkle with a pinch of salt. Toss gently until the pieces are evenly coated. Roast the squash until lightly browned and tender, about 20 minutes, stirring the squash halfway through cooking. Let the squash cool completely.

4 To assemble each salad, pour 2 tablespoons dressing into the bottom of a wide-neck quart-size Mason jar. Add half of the farro, followed by half of the squash, 2 tablespoons of the pomegranate seeds, half of the kale, half of the Brussels sprouts, 2 tablespoons of the pumpkin seeds, and 1 tablespoon of the Parmesan cheese. Repeat with another wide-neck quart-size Mason jar and the remaining ingredients. Refrigerate until ready to serve.

Recipe continues

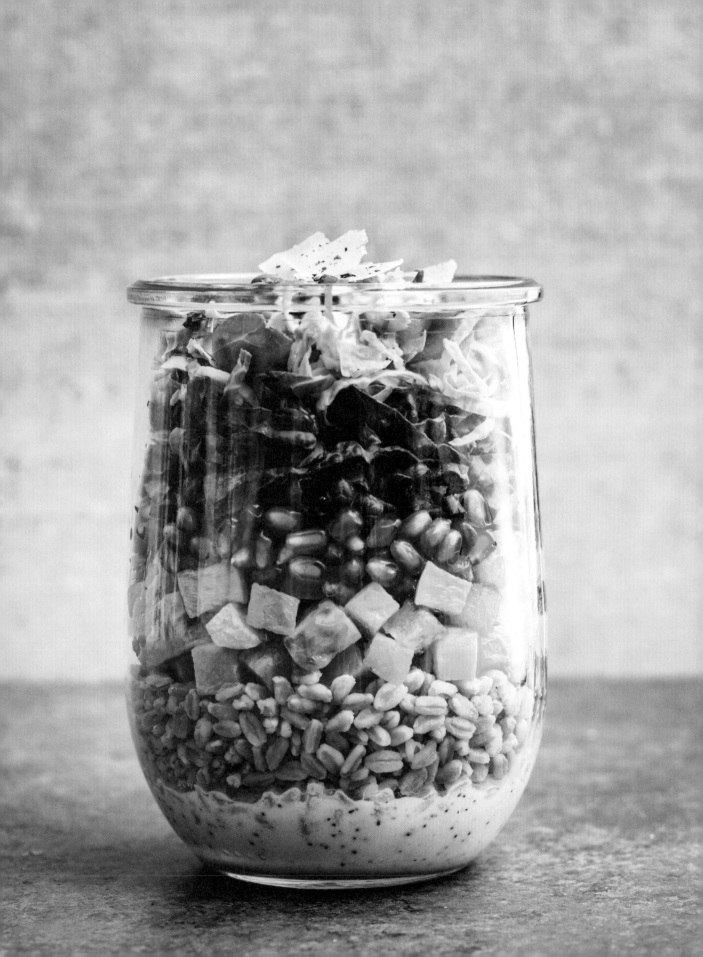

5 To serve, empty the contents of the jar into a bowl and toss well; serve immediately.

NOTE: If serving this recipe as a side salad at home, place all the prepared ingredients except for the cheese in a large serving bowl and toss to combine. Sprinkle with the cheese and serve immediately.

☺ WHAT KIDS CAN DO
Kids can help assemble the jars.

☆ MAKE AHEAD
Prep and assemble all the components, including the dressing, up to 2 days ahead of time and store in the jars in the refrigerator for a quick grab-and-go lunch.

NUTRITION INFORMATION (1 MAIN DISH SERVING):
Calories: 457 | Added sugar: ¼ teaspoon or 1g | Carbohydrates: 68g | Sodium: 634mg | Saturated fat: 5% of calories or 3g | Fiber: 15g | Protein: 16g

CHINESE CHICKEN SALAD ⬡
WITH MANDARIN VINAIGRETTE

Bright and flavorful with pops of sweet mandarin oranges, this remastered version of the popular restaurant salad hits all the right notes with no added sugar. Fresh mandarin juice subs for sugar in the dressing and adds a touch of sweetness to the roasted chicken, resulting in a light and satisfying meal.

1 Make the chicken: Arrange an oven rack about 6 inches from the broiling element and preheat the oven to broil. Line a small rimmed baking sheet with aluminum foil.

2 Combine the soy sauce, mandarin juice, garlic, and ginger in a shallow bowl. Add the chicken and toss to coat. Place the chicken on the prepared baking sheet and broil until browned and cooked through, 5 to 6 minutes per side.

3 Let the chicken cool on a cutting board for 5 to 10 minutes, then slice against the grain into bite-size pieces. If any juices collect in the pan, reserve them.

4 Make the salad: Place the chicken in a large salad bowl and add the spinach, lettuce, orange segments, green onions, half of the almonds, and half of the sesame seeds. Add the dressing and any reserved cooking juices and toss to combine. Serve, garnished with the remaining almonds and sesame seeds.

NOTES: If you can't find a mandarin orange, substitute a tangerine or a clementine.

Toasted crunchy noodles are sold in canisters in the Asian foods section of most supermarkets.

NUTRITION INFORMATION (1 SERVING WITH SESAME SEEDS):
Calories: 309 | Added sugar: 0 teaspoons or 0g | Carbohydrates: 14g |
Sodium: 332mg | Saturated fat: 6% of calories or 2g | Fiber: 4g | Protein: 32g

Ingredients

FOR THE CHICKEN

1½ tablespoons low-sodium soy sauce

1 tablespoon freshly squeezed mandarin orange juice (see Notes)

1 teaspoon finely chopped garlic

½ teaspoon peeled and finely grated fresh ginger

12 ounces boneless, skinless chicken breast, sliced through the middle to make ½-inch-thick fillets

FOR THE SALAD

4 cups baby spinach or arugula (about 4 ounces)

4 cups chopped butter lettuce (about 3 ounces) or thinly sliced cabbage

1 cup chopped mandarin orange segments (see Notes)

2 green onions, trimmed and thinly sliced

¼ cup slivered almonds, toasted

2 tablespoons toasted sesame seeds or ¼ cup broken toasted crunchy noodles (see Notes)

⅓ cup Mandarin Vinaigrette (page 193)

SERVES 4

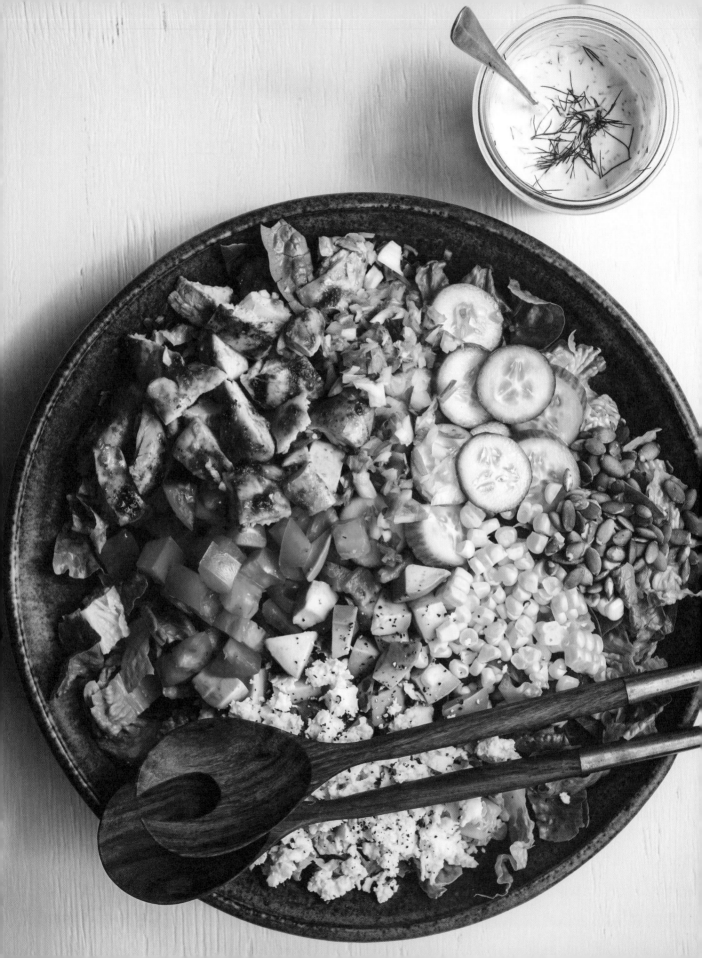

BBQ CHICKEN CHOPPED SALAD
WITH CREAMY RANCH DRESSING

OURS = ¼ TEASPOON
THEIRS = 2¼ TEASPOONS

BBQ Chicken Chopped Salad is a restaurant favorite with a sneaky amount of hidden sugar packed in what seems like a healthy choice. To drop the sugar, we use grilled chicken dressed in our low-sugar BBQ sauce, which is sweetened with peaches and cocoa powder. Smoked mozzarella amps up the flavor even more, so be sure to include it. If you have any left over, the grilled corn from our BBQ Chicken (page 96) is a great addition here.

1 Toast the pumpkin seeds in a pan over medium heat, tossing the pan a bit as they cook, until puffed and some of them pop, 5 minutes. Let cool.

2 Combine the chicken, romaine, tomatoes, cucumber, corn, and green onions in a large bowl. Add the dressing, season with the salt and pepper and toss to coat. Top with the avocado, if using, cheese, and pumpkin seeds and serve.

⚡ **QUICK TIP**
If you don't have BBQ Chicken on hand, use store-bought rotisserie chicken and toss with ¼ cup BBQ Sauce (page 185).

☆ **MAKE AHEAD**
The BBQ Chicken can be prepared the day before. It will keep, tightly wrapped in plastic wrap, in the refrigerator. This salad is also a great way to use up leftovers.

NUTRITION INFORMATION (1 SERVING):
Calories: 227 | Added sugar: ¼ teaspoon or 1g | Carbohydrates: 11g | Sodium: 479mg | Saturated fat: 14% of calories or 4g | Fiber: 3g | Protein: 22g

Ingredients

3 tablespoons hulled pumpkin seeds

2 cups diced BBQ Chicken (page 96), skin removed

6 cups chopped romaine (from 1½ to 2 hearts)

1 cup diced tomatoes

1 cup diced or sliced cucumber (preferably a seedless variety, such as Persian)

½ cup corn kernels

2 green onions, trimmed and minced

½ recipe (about ⅓ cup) Creamy Ranch Dressing (page 192)

Dash of salt and pepper

½ avocado, peeled, pitted, and diced (optional)

¼ cup shredded smoked mozzarella, regular mozzarella, queso fresco, or Monterey Jack cheese

SERVES 4

STRAWBERRY QUINOA SALAD
WITH ROASTED STRAWBERRY BALSAMIC VINAIGRETTE

OURS = 0 TEASPOONS
THEIRS = 3½ TEASPOONS

Ingredients

½ cup quinoa

1 cup low-sodium chicken broth

¼ cup chopped walnuts

1 tablespoon extra-virgin olive oil

½ teaspoon salt, plus extra as needed

5 ounces butter lettuce leaves (about 1 head), torn into bite-size pieces

1 cup sliced fresh strawberries

2 tablespoons thinly sliced green onions

¼ cup Roasted Strawberry Balsamic Vinaigrette (page 195)

1 ounce goat cheese, crumbled

Freshly ground black pepper

SERVES 2 AS A MAIN DISH OR 4 AS A SIDE DISH

Sunny strawberries add sweetness and vibrant color to this simple summer salad. Toasted quinoa provides an extra layer of nutty flavor and texture—toasting it is a step not to be skipped. Goat cheese rounds out the salad, lending a little bit of creamy deliciousness to every bite. To easily turn this salad into a more substantial main course, add hot-off-the-grill chicken as a finishing touch.

1 Preheat the oven to 400°F.

2 Rinse the quinoa thoroughly in a fine-mesh strainer. Place in a small saucepan with the chicken broth and bring to a boil over high heat. Reduce heat to low, cover, and simmer until the liquid is absorbed and the grains are fluffy, about 15 minutes.

3 While the quinoa is cooking, toast the walnuts. Spread the walnuts on a rimmed baking sheet and toast until golden brown with a nutty aroma, about 5 minutes, watching closely to prevent burning. Transfer to a plate to cool.

4 Spread the cooked quinoa on the now-empty baking sheet and toss with the olive oil and ½ teaspoon of salt. Bake until golden brown and crispy, turning occasionally, about 15 minutes. Set aside to cool.

5 Combine the lettuce, strawberries, green onions, and toasted walnuts in a large bowl. Toss with the vinaigrette, then gently fold in the goat cheese. Adjust the seasoning with a dash each of salt and pepper.

6 Spoon the salad onto plates, top with the toasted quinoa, and serve immediately.

NUTRITION INFORMATION (1 MAIN DISH SERVING):
Calories: 531 | Added sugar: 0 teaspoons or 0g | Carbohydrates: 44g | Sodium: 909mg | Saturated fat: 11% of calories or 7g | Fiber: 8g | Protein: 16g

ROMAINE AND CHERRY TOMATO SALAD
WITH MISO DRESSING

 OURS = 0 TEASPOONS
THEIRS = ¾ TEASPOON

This quick side salad delivers loads of umami flavor with very little effort and no added sugar. It's great as an extra veggie booster for Beef and Broccoli Teriyaki Bowls (page 109).

1 Whisk together the vinegar, vegetable oil, miso, sesame oil, and soy sauce in a small bowl.

2 Place the lettuce, tomatoes, and green onions in a serving bowl, add the dressing, and toss to combine. Serve immediately.

☺ **WHAT KIDS CAN DO**
Kids can whisk the salad dressing.

NUTRITION INFORMATION (1 SERVING):
Calories: 96 | Added sugar: 0 teaspoons or 0g | Carbohydrates: 5g | Sodium: 191mg | Saturated fat: 6% of calories or 1g | Fiber: 2g | Protein: 2g

Ingredients

2 tablespoons unseasoned rice vinegar

2 tablespoons vegetable oil

1 tablespoon white miso paste

½ teaspoon toasted (dark) sesame oil

½ teaspoon low-sodium soy sauce

5 cups romaine lettuce, sliced into 1-inch pieces (about 2 hearts)

1 cup cherry tomatoes, halved

2 green onions, trimmed and thinly sliced

SERVES 4 AS A SIDE DISH

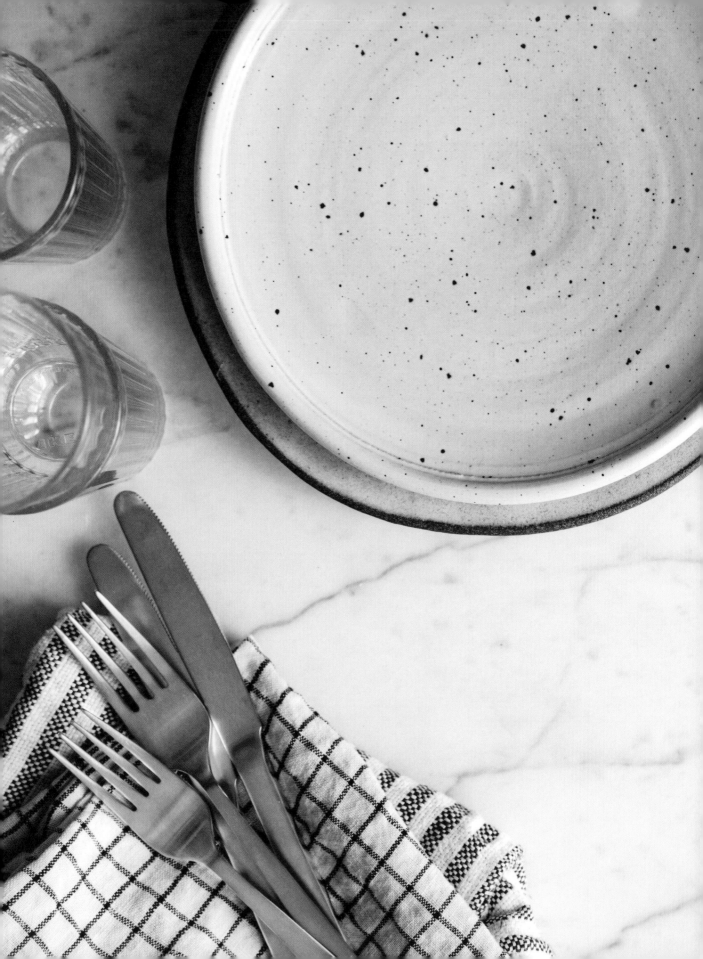

DINNERS

When it comes to dinner, it's the sauces that are the main source of added sugar. Packaged BBQ sauce, hoisin sauce, teriyaki glaze, and tomato sauce contain a significant amount of hidden added sugar that accumulates quickly in your favorite dinner dishes. That's why many of our dinner recipes make use of low-sugar (or no-added-sugar) Big Batch Sauces (see pages 185 to 189) that you can assemble ahead of time so they are ready to go when you're ready to cook. But we understand you won't always have the good fortune of advance prep, so whenever possible, we've included a Quick Tip, which allows you to make these sauces on the fly. And because we know you're busy, we've also included recipes that don't require you to make a separate sauce at all, but instead use fruits and vegetables to flavor the dish right in the pan.

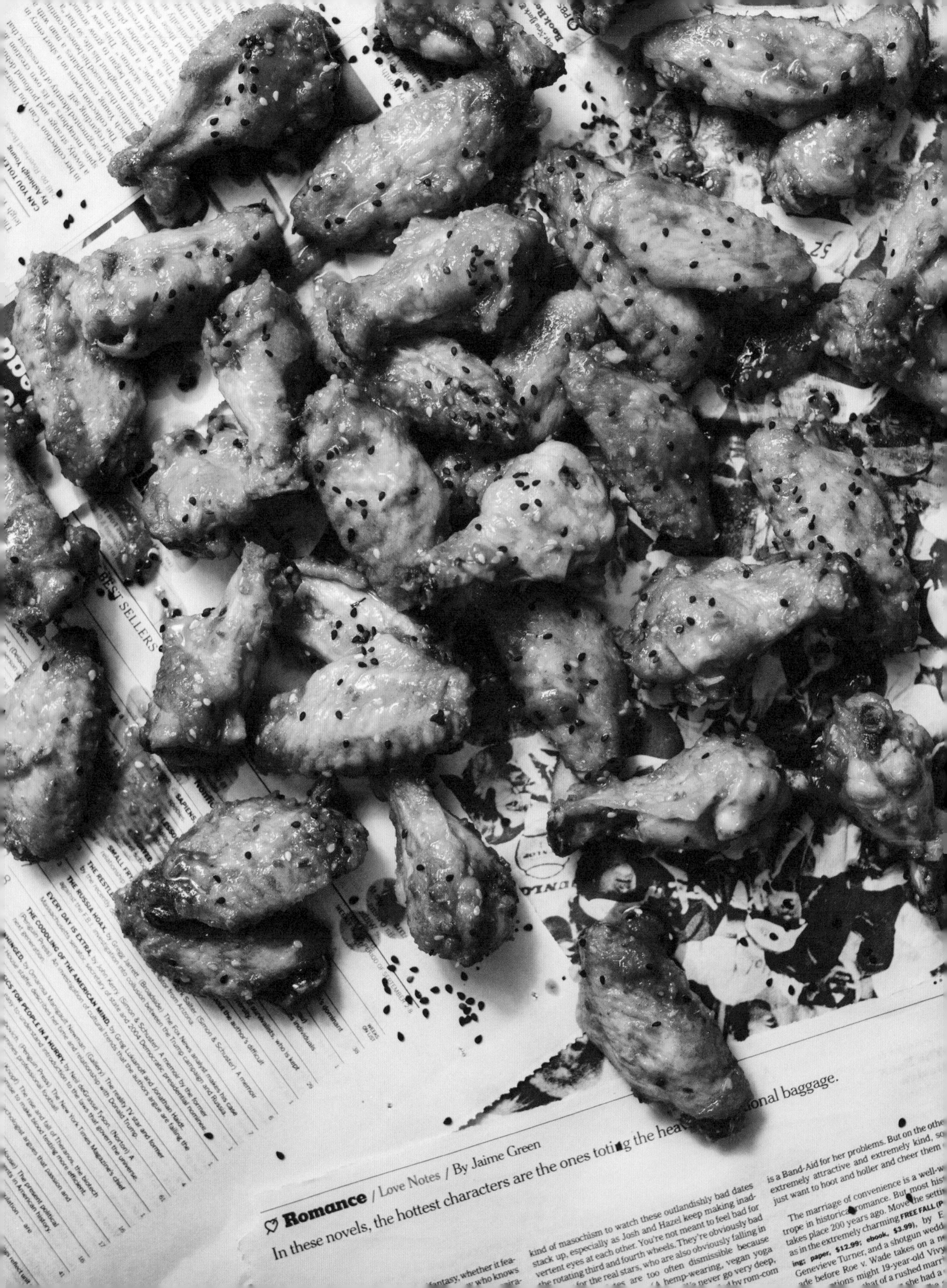
Romance / Love Notes / By Jaime Green
BEST SELLERS

OVEN-BAKED KOREAN CHICKEN WINGS

OURS = 0 TEASPOONS
THEIRS = 3¼ TEASPOONS

Unlike their batter-coated American cousins, spicy Korean fried chicken wings have a delicately crisp skin and are drenched in a mildly spicy and sweet chile paste called gochujang (go-choo-jang) sauce. This deliciously addictive condiment is the secret to the wings, but it's loaded with added sugar. Dates are the magic ingredient that help sweeten and thicken the sauces here—no added sugar required. Make 'em spicy with Sweet and Spicy Chile Sauce or mild and savory with Sweet Soy-Garlic Sauce, both of which you can mix up while the wings cook. These oven-baked wings provide a great base for either sauce to cling to.

1 Preheat the oven to 450°F and set the oven racks on the upper-middle and lower-middle positions. Line two rimmed baking sheets with aluminum foil and set a wire rack on top of each.

2 Pat the wings dry with paper towels and transfer to a large bowl. Add the oil and toss to coat. Arrange the wings on the racks atop the baking sheets, spacing them evenly apart. Sprinkle with the salt.

3 Bake until the skin is crisp and golden, about 45 minutes, turning the pieces over every 15 minutes.

4 In a medium bowl, toss half of the wings with half of the sauce until evenly coated. Transfer to a serving platter. Repeat with the remaining wings and sauce. Serve immediately.

Ingredients

4 pounds chicken wings, separated into flats and drumettes, wing tips removed

2 tablespoons vegetable oil

2 teaspoons kosher salt

1 recipe Sweet and Spicy Chile Sauce (page 94) or Sweet Soy-Garlic Sauce (page 95)

SERVES 8

NUTRITION INFORMATION (4 OR 5 PIECES WITH SWEET AND SPICY CHILE SAUCE):
Calories: 515 | Added sugar: 0 teaspoons or 0g | Carbohydrates: 8g | Sodium: 742mg | Saturated fat: 15% of calories or 9g | Fiber: 1g | Protein: 41g

Sweet and Spicy Chile Sauce ⬡

OURS: 0 TEASPOONS
THEIRS: 4¼ TEASPOONS

Ingredients

2 ounces Deglet Noor
dates, pitted
(about 8 dates)

2 cups boiling water

1 teaspoon vegetable oil

1 teaspoon peeled and
finely grated fresh
ginger

2 cloves garlic, peeled and
minced

2 tablespoons low-sodium
soy sauce

2 tablespoons sriracha

1 tablespoon tomato paste

1 tablespoon white miso
paste

1 teaspoon unseasoned
rice vinegar

1 teaspoon toasted (dark)
sesame oil

1 tablespoon toasted
sesame seeds

MAKES ABOUT ¾ CUP

This spicy sauce is a no-added-sugar version of traditional gochujang sauce. It's sweetened with dates, and the kick comes from a touch of sriracha.

1 Place the dates in a small bowl and cover with the boiling water. Let sit for 10 minutes. Drain, reserving ¼ cup of the soaking liquid. Set aside.

2 Heat the oil in a small skillet over medium heat. Add the ginger and garlic and cook until fragrant, about 1 minute.

3 Transfer the ginger and garlic to a blender, add the reserved soaking liquid and then the dates, soy sauce, sriracha, tomato paste, miso paste, vinegar, and sesame oil. Blend until smooth and no chunks of dates remain, about 2 minutes, stopping the blender to scrape the side of the container as needed.

4 Pour the sauce into a jar or airtight container and stir in the sesame seeds to finish.

☆ **MAKE AHEAD**
The sauce will keep, covered, in the refrigerator for up to 1 week.

NUTRITION INFORMATION (2 TABLESPOONS):
Calories: 68 | Added sugar: 0 teaspoons or 0g | Carbohydrates: 11g | Sodium: 425mg | Saturated fat: 4% of calories or <1g | Fiber: 2g | Protein: 1g

Sweet Soy-Garlic Sauce

OURS: 0 TEASPOONS
THEIRS: 6¾ TEASPOONS

Kids may prefer a milder flavor on their wings, which is where this garlicky soy sauce comes into play. Dates add natural sweetness, and crushed red pepper flakes lend just enough spice to keep things interesting. If you prefer a milder sauce, feel free to omit the red pepper flakes.

1 Place the dates in a small bowl and cover with the boiling water. Let sit for 10 minutes. Drain, reserving ¼ cup of the soaking liquid. Set aside.

2 Heat the oil in a small skillet over medium heat. Add the ginger and garlic and cook until fragrant, about 1 minute.

3 Transfer the ginger and garlic to a blender, add the reserved soaking liquid, and then add the dates, soy sauce, vinegar, sesame oil, and red pepper flakes, if using. Blend until smooth and no chunks of dates remain, about 2 minutes, stopping the blender to scrape the side of the container as needed. Pour the sauce into a jar or airtight container.

☆ **MAKE AHEAD**
The sauce will keep, covered, in the refrigerator for up to 1 week.

Ingredients

1½ ounces Deglet Noor dates, pitted (about 6 dates)

2 cups boiling water

1 teaspoon vegetable oil

1 teaspoon peeled and finely grated fresh ginger

2 cloves garlic, peeled and minced

¼ cup low-sodium soy sauce

1 tablespoon unseasoned rice vinegar

2 teaspoons toasted (dark) sesame oil

¼ teaspoon crushed red pepper flakes (optional)

MAKES ABOUT ¾ CUP

NUTRITION INFORMATION (2 TABLESPOONS):
Calories: 48 | Added sugar: 0 teaspoons or 0g | Carbohydrates: 7g | Sodium: 356mg | Saturated fat: 5% of calories or <1g | Fiber: 1g | Protein: 1g

BBQ CHICKEN
WITH GRILLED CORN SALAD

OURS: ¼ TEASPOON
THEIRS: 2 TEASPOONS

Ingredients

FOR THE CHICKEN

4 bone-in, skin-on chicken
thighs or 2 whole legs,
with the drumsticks
and thighs divided
(1½ pounds)
½ teaspoon kosher salt
Freshly ground black
pepper
1 tablespoon vegetable oil
¼ cup BBQ Sauce
(page 185), plus extra
for serving

FOR THE SALAD

3 ears corn, shucked and
boiled (see Note)
2 cups arugula
1 large tomato, cored and
chopped into ¼-inch
dice
1 green onion, trimmed
and thinly sliced
2 tablespoons extra-virgin
olive oil, plus extra as
needed
2 teaspoons white wine
vinegar or 1 teaspoon
balsamic vinegar, plus
extra as needed
Dash of salt and pepper

SERVES 4

BBQ chicken is a summertime cookout classic, but added sugar can rack up quickly when you use jarred BBQ sauce. Add to that the hidden sugar in your salad dressing and a side of generously sweetened baked beans, and suddenly dinner isn't so healthy anymore. The remastered BBQ Sauce (page 185) we use here saves the day, slashing added sugar to one quarter of a teaspoon. And our tasty Boston Baked Beans (page 97) offer a delicious low-sugar assist. While the chicken cooks slowly over indirect heat, you can grill the corn until it's nice and toasty. If you don't like arugula, substitute chopped romaine or a handful of chopped fresh basil or cilantro.

1 Preheat the grill to indirect medium heat (350°F to 450°F). If using a gas grill, place half of the burners on medium, leaving the other half of the grill unheated. If using a charcoal grill, move the coals over to one side so there's a space on the grill that's not directly over the coals.

2 Place the chicken on a rimmed baking sheet or in a large bowl. Season the chicken on both sides with the salt and pepper, then drizzle with the vegetable oil and toss to coat. Grill the chicken bone side down over indirect heat for about 40 minutes, until it has reached at least 160°F in the thickest part (test it with an instant-read thermometer).

3 While the chicken cooks over indirect heat on the grill, cook the corn over direct heat for 7 to 10 minutes, turning it so it browns on all sides. Keep the grill covered as much as you can while it cooks. Transfer the corn to a cutting board and let cool.

4 Move the chicken pieces over the flame and cook, turning once, until browned all over, about 3 minutes per side (move the pieces away from any flare-ups, which will cause burning). Brush the ¼ cup sauce on the chicken, coating each piece all over, and cook to sear the sauce onto the skin, 2 minutes per side. Remove from the grill and let rest for 5 to 10 minutes.

5 Use a sharp knife to slice the corn kernels off the cobs and into a medium bowl. Add the arugula, tomato, green onion, olive oil, vinegar, and salt and pepper, and toss to combine.

6 Serve the chicken with the salad and extra sauce on the side (warm it in a small saucepan over low heat if you wish).

NOTE: To boil the corn, bring a large pot of water to a boil, add the corn and cook until tender, 5 to 6 minutes. Drain well.

Boston Baked Beans

OURS = 1 TEASPOON
THEIRS = 2 TO 2¾ TEASPOONS

Pureed ripe pear is the secret ingredient that provides most of the sweetness in this simplified, smoky take on the classic. It's the perfect side dish for summer cookouts.

1 Preheat the oven to 350°F.

2 Cook the bacon in a Dutch oven over medium-high heat, stirring occasionally, until crisp, about 5 minutes. Using a slotted spoon, transfer the bacon to a bowl.

3 Add the onions to the pot, reduce the heat to medium, and cover. Cook until very soft and caramelized, about 20 minutes, uncovering to stir occasionally and adding ½ cup water halfway through cooking.

4 Meanwhile, place the pear and ¼ cup water in a food processor or blender and process until smooth.

5 Return the bacon to the pot and stir in the beans, 1 cup water, the pear puree, molasses, paprika, mustard, salt, and pepper. Bring to a simmer over medium-high heat.

6 Transfer the pot to the oven and bake the beans, uncovered, until thickened, about 30 minutes. Serve hot.

Ingredients

2 slices bacon, diced
2 large sweet onions, peeled and diced (about 4 cups)
1 very ripe Bartlett pear, cored and diced (skin left on)
2 cans (15.5 ounces each) navy beans or Great Northern beans, rinsed and drained
2 tablespoons molasses (not blackstrap)
1 teaspoon smoked paprika
1 teaspoon dry mustard
½ teaspoon salt
½ teaspoon freshly ground black pepper

SERVES 8

CHINESE CHICKEN LETTUCE CUPS

 OURS = ¼ TEASPOON
THEIRS: 1¼ TEASPOONS

Ingredients

1 cup medium-grain white or brown rice

2 tablespoons vegetable oil

1 medium zucchini, trimmed and cut into small dice

1 large red bell pepper, stemmed, seeded, and cut into small dice

2 cloves garlic, peeled and finely chopped

¼ teaspoon salt

¼ teaspoon crushed red pepper flakes (optional)

1 pound lean ground chicken or turkey

¼ cup Chinese Hoisin Sauce (page 187)

2 green onions, trimmed and minced

8 large butter lettuce leaves

Sriracha, for serving (optional)

SERVES 4

This easy dinner is based on a classic recipe for Chinese lettuce wraps. It's super fun for kids to eat because no forks are required! Our low-sugar Chinese Hoisin Sauce adds plenty of sweetness with very little added sugar.

1 Cook the rice according to package directions. When done, remove the rice from the heat and let it steam, covered, in the pot.

2 Heat 1 tablespoon of the oil in a wok or large skillet over medium-high heat and add the zucchini and bell pepper and half of the garlic. Season with ⅛ teaspoon of the salt and stir-fry until the vegetables are crisp-tender, 4 to 5 minutes. Transfer to a small bowl.

3 Add the remaining 1 tablespoon oil and the remaining garlic to the pan with the red pepper flakes, if using, and swirl to coat the pan. Add the chicken and stir-fry over high heat, breaking up the meat as you go, until cooked through, 3 to 5 minutes. Add half of the hoisin sauce and stir-fry for 30 seconds.

4 Reduce the heat to medium and add the cooked vegetables, green onions, and remaining hoisin sauce to the pan. Gently toss over medium heat to incorporate the ingredients. Season with the remaining ⅛ teaspoon of salt and remove from the heat.

5 Place the rice, lettuce leaves, and stir-fry on the table. Have everyone scoop a spoonful of rice and stir-fry into each lettuce cup as they eat, topping with a touch of sriracha if they like.

⚡ QUICK TIP
To make a quick sub for the hoisin sauce, in a small bowl combine ¼ cup low-sodium soy sauce, 1 tablespoon unseasoned rice vinegar, 2 teaspoons toasted (dark) sesame oil, 2 teaspoons peeled and minced fresh ginger, ¼ teaspoon Chinese five-spice powder, ¼ teaspoon crushed red pepper flakes, and ⅛ teaspoon ground black pepper.

☺ WHAT KIDS CAN DO
Kids can separate and wash the lettuce leaves.

☆ MAKE AHEAD
To save time, chop the zucchini and bell pepper 1 day ahead and store in an airtight container in the refrigerator.

NUTRITION INFORMATION (1 SERVING):
Calories: 427 | Added sugar: ¼ teaspoon or 1g | Carbohydrates: 46g | Sodium: 860mg | Saturated fat: 7% of calories or 3g | Fiber: 3g | Protein: 22g

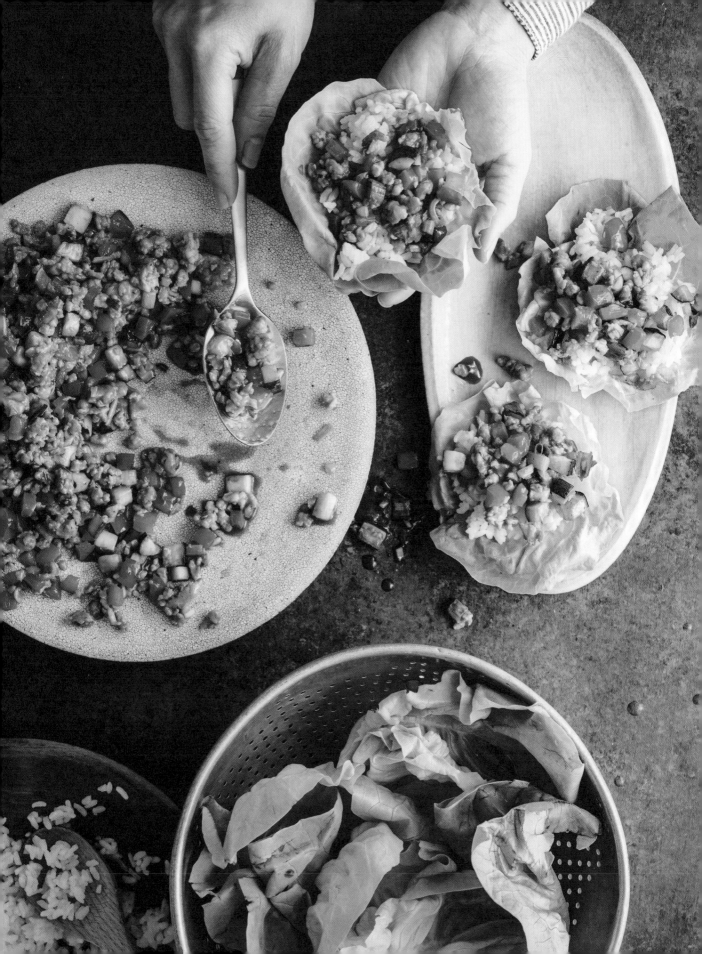

CITRUS CHICKEN STIR-FRY
WITH GREEN BEANS

OURS = 0 TEASPOONS
THEIRS: 6¼ TEASPOONS

Ingredients

1 cup short- or medium-grain brown rice

¼ cup low-sodium soy sauce

3 tablespoons freshly squeezed tangerine or orange juice

3 tablespoons freshly squeezed lemon juice

1 tablespoon toasted (dark) sesame oil

1 teaspoon peeled and finely grated fresh ginger

1 pound boneless, skinless chicken breast or thigh meat, cut into 2 x ¼-inch slices

1 teaspoon cornstarch

¼ cup slivered almonds

1 tablespoon vegetable oil

8 ounces green beans, trimmed and cut into 2-inch pieces (about 2 cups)

Sriracha or other hot sauce, for serving (optional)

SERVES 4

The restaurant version of this popular dish is battered, fried, and loaded with sweet syrupy sauce. Tangerine juice and freshly grated ginger are used here to create a fresh citrus flavor reminiscent of the original without any added sugar. Use chicken thighs instead of breasts for more tender bites.

1 Bring 2 quarts water to a boil. Add the rice and cook according to the package directions. Drain, then return to the pot right away, cover, and let steam for 5 to 10 minutes before serving.

2 Combine the soy sauce, tangerine juice, lemon juice, sesame oil, and ginger in a small measuring cup. Stir well. Place the chicken in a medium bowl and toss with 2 tablespoons of the sauce.

3 Add the cornstarch and 1 tablespoon cold water to the remaining sauce, stirring well to dissolve the cornstarch.

4 Heat a wok or large skillet over medium heat. Add the almonds and toss until lightly toasted, about 4 minutes. Transfer the nuts to a plate and set aside to cool.

5 Increase the heat to medium-high, then add the oil and swirl to coat the pan. Add the chicken mixture and stir-fry until mostly cooked through, 5 minutes.

6 Add the green beans and stir-fry until tender, 2 to 3 minutes. During the last minute, add the remaining sauce and cook until the sauce thickens. Serve hot, over the rice, sprinkled with the almonds and with the hot sauce on the side, if using.

☺ WHAT KIDS CAN DO
Kids can remove the stems from the green beans and juice the tangerines and lemons.

☆ MAKE AHEAD
The chicken can marinate, tightly wrapped in plastic wrap, in the refrigerator for 1 day.

NUTRITION INFORMATION (1 SERVING):
Calories: 463 | Added sugar: 0 teaspoons or 0g | Carbohydrates: 49g | Sodium: 996mg | Saturated fat: 6% of calories or 3g | Fiber: 4g | Protein: 25g

VIETNAMESE CHICKEN NOODLE SOUP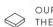

OURS: 0 TEASPOONS
THEIRS: ¼ TEASPOON

Sweet onion and Asian pear, combined with ginger and fragrant spices, come together in this simplified version of traditional Vietnamese chicken noodle soup. Restaurant versions of this dish contain rock sugar to sweeten the broth. Asian pear does the trick here, sweetening without the need for added sugar. We've also reduced the fish sauce—an essential ingredient in the broth but high in sodium—and added low-sodium soy sauce to round out the flavors.

1 Make the broth: Heat the oil in a large stock pot or Dutch oven over high heat. Add the onion, pear, and ginger and cook until slightly charred and fragrant, about 5 minutes. Reduce the heat if they start to smoke.

2 Add the coriander seeds, if using, and the cloves, star anise pods, cinnamon sticks, and chicken thighs to the pot along with 8 cups water, the fish sauce, and the soy sauce. Bring the mixture to a boil over high heat, then reduce the heat, cover, and simmer, skimming occasionally, until the meat is tender and falling off the bone, about 1½ hours.

3 Transfer the chicken to a cutting board and discard the skin and bones. Using a fork, gently pull apart the meat into large chunks and set aside.

4 Pour the broth through a fine-mesh strainer into a medium pot and discard the solids. Skim off any remaining fat from the surface of the broth. Add the meat to the pot and heat until warmed through, 3 to 5 minutes.

5 To serve, portion the noodles into six bowls. Top evenly with the chicken and broth. Add the basil, bean sprouts, and cilantro and finish with a squeeze of lime juice and a touch of hoisin sauce if you like.

NOTE: Fresh and dried noodles vary in weight, so follow the package directions to gauge serving size.

⚡ QUICK TIP
This recipe can also be made in a pressure cooker. After adding the liquid in Step 2, seal the pressure cooker and cook on high for 20 minutes.

NUTRITION INFORMATION (1 SERVING):
Calories: 341 | Added sugar: 0 teaspoons or 0g | Carbohydrates: 45g | Sodium: 923mg | Saturated fat: 5% of calories or 2g | Fiber: 4g | Protein: 17g

Ingredients

FOR THE BROTH
2 tablespoons vegetable oil
1 large sweet onion, peeled and cut into quarters
1 large Asian pear, peeled, cored, and cut into large chunks
5 large coins peeled fresh ginger
1 teaspoon coriander seeds (optional)
5 whole cloves
4 star anise pods
2 cinnamon sticks
1½ pounds bone-in, skin-on chicken thighs
2 tablespoons fish sauce
2 tablespoons low-sodium soy sauce

FOR SERVING
6 servings pho rice noodles, preferably fresh (see Note), prepared according to package directions
4 fresh basil sprigs, stems removed
2 cups mung bean sprouts
1 small bunch fresh cilantro, stems removed
2 limes, each cut into 4 wedges
Chinese Hoisin Sauce (page 187) or sriracha (optional)

SERVES 6

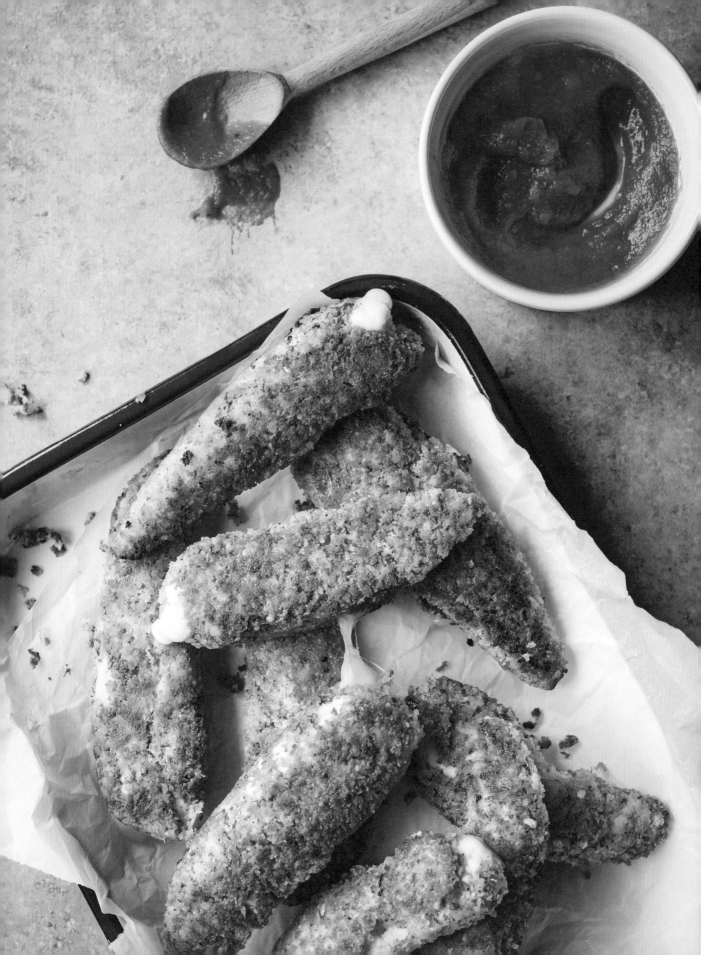

STUFFED CHICKEN PARMESAN STRIPS
WITH 5-MINUTE MARINARA DIPPING SAUCE

OURS = ¼ TEASPOON
THEIRS = ¾ TEASPOON

Using uniformly sized chicken breast tenders (the hanging strip of meat located on the underside of each chicken breast) and string cheese reduces the prep work in putting together this kid-friendly meal. Look for chicken tenders in the grocery store meat department, or ask your butcher for them. Ground flaxseed takes the place of all-purpose flour for an extra boost of nutrition. A quick pan-fry coupled with a few minutes of baking ensures that the breading is browned and crisp, the chicken is cooked through, and the cheese is melted to perfection.

1 Preheat the oven to 400°F. Line a rimmed baking sheet with aluminum foil and coat it with cooking spray.

2 Whisk together the flaxseed and salt in a shallow bowl or pie plate. In another bowl or pie plate, whisk together the panko and Parmesan. In a third bowl, whisk together the eggs and 1 tablespoon water. Set aside.

3 Cut each string cheese stick in half crosswise and then again in half lengthwise to yield a total of 8 pieces. Set aside.

4 Insert a paring knife through the middle of one end of a chicken tender. Gently cut a pocket through the length of the tender, leaving both sides and the other end of the tender intact. Repeat with the remaining chicken tenders. Insert one piece of string cheese into each pocket.

5 Working with one stuffed chicken tender at a time, dredge the chicken in the flaxseed mixture, shaking off any excess. Dip the chicken into the egg wash, allowing any excess to drip off, then coat with the panko mixture, pressing gently so the crumbs adhere. Transfer to a large plate and repeat with the remaining tenders.

6 Heat the oil in a large nonstick skillet over medium-high heat until shimmering. Arrange the tenders in the skillet in a single layer and cook until golden brown and crisp on the first side, about 3 minutes. Flip the tenders over, moving the pieces around if necessary, and cook until golden brown on the second side, about 3 minutes.

7 Transfer the tenders to the prepared baking sheet. Bake until the cheese is melted and the

Ingredients

Nonstick cooking spray
⅓ cup ground flaxseed
¼ teaspoon salt
¾ cup panko breadcrumbs
¼ cup grated Parmesan cheese
2 large eggs
2 sticks part-skim mozzarella string cheese, unwrapped
8 chicken breast tenders (2 ounces each)
3 tablespoons extra-virgin olive oil
5-Minute Marinara Dipping Sauce (page 104), for serving

SERVES 4

chicken is cooked through, 5 to 7 minutes.

8 Serve immediately with the dipping sauce.

⚡ **QUICK TIP**
Depending on the size of the chicken tenders, it may be a little tricky to tuck the cheese inside. You can slice the cheese in half again to make it easier.

NUTRITION INFORMATION (2 PIECES WITH ¼ CUP SAUCE):
Calories: 516 | Added sugar: ¼ teaspoon or 1g | Carbohydrates: 25g | Sodium: 708mg | Saturated fat: 11% of calories or 6g | Fiber: 5g | Protein: 41g

5-Minute Marinara Dipping Sauce ⬡

OURS = 0 TEASPOONS
THEIRS = ¼ TEASPOON

Ingredients

1 tablespoon extra-virgin olive oil
1 teaspoon minced garlic
1 can (15 ounces) no-salt-added tomato sauce
¼ teaspoon dried oregano
¼ teaspoon salt

MAKES 1¼ CUPS

Homemade marinara sauce typically requires at least half an hour of simmering, while prepared versions can contain a fair amount of added sugar. This speedy version takes less than 5 minutes to make—about the same amount of time required to heat up a jar of store-bought sauce. It makes just the right amount to pair with our Stuffed Chicken Parmesan Strips (page 103).

Heat the oil in a small saucepan over medium heat. Add the garlic and cook until fragrant, about 30 seconds, stirring frequently. Add the tomato sauce, oregano, and salt and bring to a simmer. Remove from the heat. Cover and keep warm until ready to serve.

⭐ **MAKE AHEAD**
The sauce will keep in an airtight container in the refrigerator for 1 week.

NUTRITION INFORMATION (¼ CUP):
Calories: 34 | Added sugar: 0 teaspoons or 0g | Carbohydrates: 4g | Sodium: 90mg | Saturated fat: 8% of calories or <1g | Fiber: 1g | Protein: 1g

BBQ PULLED PORK SLIDERS
WITH TANGY BUTTERMILK APPLE SLAW

OURS: 1¼ TEASPOONS
THEIRS: 3½ TO 6¾ TEASPOONS

BBQ pulled pork sliders are a game-day favorite. The secret to dropping the sugar in these is using ripe nectarines and cocoa powder to sweeten the sauce. Apples in the slaw add extra sweetness and delicious crunch. This recipe makes a big batch, so you'll comfortably please a crowd or have leftovers for a quick weekday lunch. You can cook the pork in a 6-quart slow cooker or in the oven (see the Variation on page 106), depending on your preference. Serve the slaw on the side or inside the sliders.

1 Rub the pork with the spice mix, covering all the surfaces well.

2 Heat a large skillet over medium-high heat. Add the oil and heat until hot but not smoking. Swirl to coat the pan. Add the pork and brown on all sides, a few minutes per side. Watch closely so the spice coating doesn't burn.

3 Transfer the pork to a slow cooker, then pour the BBQ sauce and chicken broth around the sides. Cover and cook until the meat is very tender and can be pulled apart with a fork, on high heat for 3 to 4 hours or on low heat for 6 to 8 hours.

4 Finish the pork: Remove the pork from the cooker and transfer to a cutting board. Spoon the oil off the top of the sauce. Shred the pork with two forks, removing any big chunks of fat, then return the meat to the sauce and stir together gently, adding white vinegar and salt to taste. Keep warm.

5 Make the slaw: Whisk together the buttermilk, olive oil, cider vinegar, ¼ teaspoon salt, and ⅛ teaspoon pepper in a large bowl. Add the cabbage, carrots, apple, green onions, and cilantro, if using, and toss together. Season with more salt and pepper to taste.

6 Make the sliders: Scoop some of the pork into each bun and either top with some of the slaw or serve the slaw on the side. Serve immediately with the hot sauce, if using.

Recipe continues

Ingredients

2½ pounds boneless pork shoulder or pork butt, untrussed, thick outer fat removed

1½ tablespoons BBQ Spice Mix (page 185)

2 tablespoons vegetable oil

2 cups BBQ Sauce (page 185)

1 cup low-sodium chicken broth

White vinegar

Fine sea salt

2 tablespoons buttermilk or plain whole milk yogurt

2 tablespoons olive oil

1 tablespoon apple cider vinegar

Freshly ground black pepper

3 cups thinly sliced green or red cabbage

1 cup shredded or matchstick carrots

1 red apple, cored (skin on) and cut into matchsticks

2 tablespoons minced green onions

Fresh cilantro leaves (optional)

10 large or 20 small slider buns, split, buttered, and warmed

Hot sauce, for serving (optional)

SERVES 10

VARIATION: To make the pork in the oven, preheat the oven to 300°F. Sear the spice-rubbed pork in a Dutch oven as directed in Step 2, then remove the pork to a plate and drain off the oil. Return the pork to the pot and pour the BBQ sauce and chicken broth around the sides. Bring to a simmer over medium heat, then cover and place in the oven. Roast until the meat is very tender and can be pulled apart with a fork, flipping once after 1½ hours, 3 to 4 hours total. Proceed with the recipe from Step 4.

⚡ **QUICK TIP**
If you don't have time to make the BBQ Sauce in advance, use the Quick Tip on page 185 and reduce the chicken broth in this recipe to ½ cup.

☺ **WHAT KIDS CAN DO**
Little chefs can whisk the dressing for the slaw.

☆ **MAKE AHEAD**
You can make the slaw up to 3 hours ahead. It will keep in an airtight container in the refrigerator until you're ready to serve.

NUTRITION INFORMATION (1 LARGE SLIDER):
Calories: 417 | Added sugar: 1¼ teaspoons or 5g | Carbohydrates: 37g | Sodium: 734mg | Saturated fat: 10% of calories or 5g | Fiber: 4g | Protein: 24g

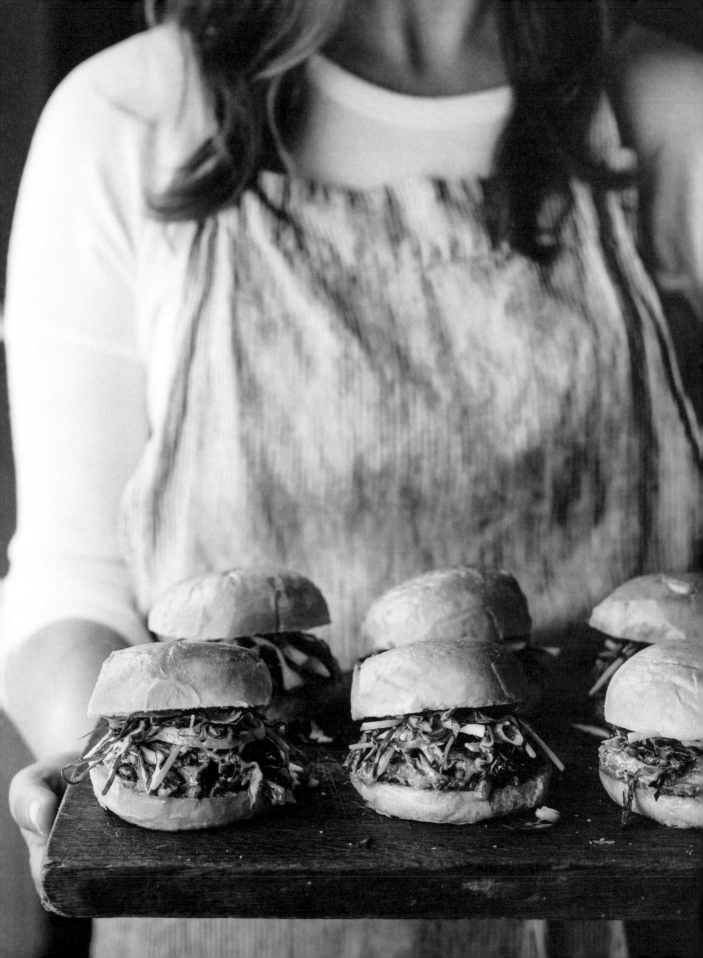

SWEET AND STICKY CHINESE BBQ PORK ROAST (*CHAR SIU*) ⊗

OURS = 0 TEASPOONS*
THEIRS = 1 TEASPOON

Ingredients

½ cup Chinese Hoisin
    Sauce (page 187)
2 tablespoons tomato
    paste
½ teaspoon kosher salt
3 pounds boneless pork
    shoulder, trussed

SERVES 10

This low-sugar version of Chinese BBQ pork (*char siu*) still has the shiny red coating and juicy flavor that you'd expect from this classic dish, but with a fraction of the sugar. Make it on a weekend when you have time to let the meat slow-roast in the oven. Serve a crowd or save yourself some cooking time and work tender, tasty slices of pork into dishes all week long. Char siu is a great addition to a steamy bowl of noodles or chopped into cubes and tossed into a quick fried rice, like Chinese BBQ Pork Fried Rice (page 78). It's always good to cook pork shoulder to an internal temperature of at least 160°F for the best texture, so use your meat thermometer. Serve it with rice and lightly sautéed leafy greens like bok choy or Chinese broccoli.

1 Whisk together the hoisin sauce, tomato paste, and salt in a small bowl. Place the pork in a resealable plastic bag and add the sauce. Seal the bag and turn the pork in the sauce to coat evenly. Marinate overnight in the refrigerator.

2 When ready to roast the pork, preheat the oven to 300°F. Line a roasting pan with aluminum foil and set a rack inside the pan. Set the pork on the rack.

3 Roast until the meat is crispy on the edges and browned, and the internal temperature reaches at least 160°F (and as much as 170°F), 2½ to 3 hours.

4 Cover with aluminum foil and let rest at least 10 minutes before thinly slicing the meat against the grain. Serve immediately.

☆ **MAKE AHEAD**
The cooked pork will keep, tightly wrapped in plastic wrap, in the refrigerator for up to 1 week.

NUTRITION INFORMATION (ABOUT 2½ OUNCES):
Calories: 318 | Added sugar: 0 teaspoons or 0g | Carbohydrates: 3g | Sodium: 661mg | Saturated fat: 23% of calories or 8g | Fiber: 0g | Protein: 24g

*Negligible

BEEF AND BROCCOLI TERIYAKI BOWLS

 OURS: ¾ TEASPOON
THEIRS = 1½ TEASPOONS

Thinly slicing beef against the grain and tossing it lightly in cornstarch makes it very tender in this easy stir-fry. Pineapple Teriyaki Glaze lends a naturally sweet and salty flavor and helps slash the added sugar by half of what you'd typically find in a packaged frozen dinner. Brown rice is highly nutritious, but some kids may take time to warm up to its flavor and texture. The natural oils in brown rice can make it turn rancid easily and taste bitter, especially to kids. Be sure to buy fresh brown rice and keep it in the refrigerator. Using more of a pasta-cooking method and letting the rice steam in the pot for a while before serving also makes it tastier.

1 Bring 2 quarts water to a boil. Add the rice and boil according to the package directions, then drain. Return to the pot right away, cover, and let steam for 5 to 10 minutes before serving.

2 Meanwhile, place 1 teaspoon cornstarch in a large bowl, add the beef, and toss to coat. Place the remaining 2 teaspoons cornstarch in a small bowl, add ¼ cup water, and stir to combine.

3 Heat 1 tablespoon of the oil in a wok or large skillet over high heat. When it's hot, toss in the baby broccoli, stir-frying until bright green and wilted, 1 to 2 minutes.

Add 2 tablespoons water, cover, and steam until crisp-tender, 1 to 2 minutes more. Remove from the pan to a plate.

4 Add the remaining 1 tablespoon oil to the pan, then toss in the beef mixture, stir-frying until tender and lightly browned, about 4 minutes.

5 Return the baby broccoli to the pan and add the teriyaki glaze. Bring to a simmer, then stir in the cornstarch slurry. Return to a simmer and let cook until the sauce has thickened, about 1 minute. Stir to coat everything in the pan.

Recipe continues

Ingredients

1 cup short- or medium-grain brown rice

3 teaspoons cornstarch

12 ounces flank steak or top sirloin beef, sliced very thinly against the grain into 2 x 1 x ⅛-inch strips

2 tablespoons vegetable oil

2 bunches baby broccoli, cut into 2-inch lengths, or about 4 cups broccoli florets

½ cup Pineapple Teriyaki Glaze (page 186)

2 teaspoons toasted sesame seeds, for garnish

2 tablespoons thinly sliced green onion, for garnish (optional)

SERVES 4

6 Scoop the brown rice into bowls and top with the teriyaki beef mixture. Serve immediately, sprinkled with sesame seeds and green onion, if using, to garnish.

VARIATION: You can also make this recipe with a 14-ounce package of firm tofu in place of the beef. Drain and cut into 1-inch cubes, then let drain again in a strainer briefly before treating it the same way as you would the beef in the recipe, gently tossing it in the cornstarch and cooking it for 3 to 4 minutes.

QUICK TIP
Using frozen precooked brown rice instead of fresh makes this dish come together in a snap. Of course, you can serve this dish with short- or medium-grain white rice, too.

NUTRITION INFORMATION (1 SERVING):
Calories: 424 | Added sugar: ¾ teaspoon or 3g | Carbohydrates: 53g | Sodium: 520mg | Saturated fat: 4% of calories or 2g | Fiber: 3g | Protein: 27g

PINEAPPLE TERIYAKI SHORT RIBS

OURS = ¾ TEASPOON
THEIRS = 6½ TEASPOONS

This recipe for braised Asian-style short ribs comes together faster if you have a batch of Pineapple Teriyaki Glaze (page 186) ready to go. Use it to replace the ingredients you combine with the broth in Step 1. It's best to cook the ribs one day ahead and refrigerate them, which allows you to remove the fat more easily, making the stew not only healthier but tastier. We like to make these in a slow cooker for ease, but they are just as delicious prepared in the oven. Serve with rice or over a pile of mashed potatoes (even better if they're flavored with wasabi!) and sautéed bok choy or Chinese broccoli.

1 Combine the soy sauce, sake, pineapple, brown sugar, garlic, ginger, and broth in a slow cooker and mix until the sugar is dissolved.

2 Heat a skillet over medium-high heat. When the pan is hot, add the oil and heat until hot but not smoking. Swirl to coat the pan. Season the short ribs with salt, then add to the pan and brown on all sides, about 2 minutes per side.

3 Place the seared meat in the slow cooker. Top with the carrots and onion. Cover and cook until the meat is tender, on high heat for 4 to 5 hours or on low heat for 8 to 10 hours.

4 Using a large spoon, scoop off the clear fat from the top of the stew and discard it.

5 Remove the short ribs from the slow cooker and discard the bones, if using bone-in ribs, then pull the meat apart into bite-size chunks. Set aside.

6 Using a fine-mesh strainer set over a large pot, strain the broth (discard the carrots and onions). Add the meat to the broth and reheat on low heat until warmed through, 5 minutes.

7 Serve the meat garnished with the green onion and togarashi spice, if using.

NOTE: Togarashi is a seven-spice blend commonly used in Japan. It can be used to top soups and rice or as a seasoning for grilling meats. It can be found in most well-stocked grocery stores or online.

Recipe continues

Ingredients

½ cup plus 2 tablespoons low-sodium soy sauce

½ cup sake

½ cup finely chopped fresh pineapple or drained crushed pineapple (canned in juice)

2½ tablespoons packed light brown sugar

2 teaspoons chopped garlic

½ teaspoon peeled and finely grated fresh ginger

4 cups low-sodium beef broth

2 tablespoons vegetable oil

2½ pounds boneless or 3½ pounds bone-in beef short ribs, fat trimmed

½ teaspoon kosher salt

2 cups carrot wedges or large chunks

2 cups onion chunks (about 1½ large peeled onions)

Thinly sliced green onion or chopped fresh cilantro, for garnish

Togarashi spice, for garnish (optional; see Note)

SERVES 10

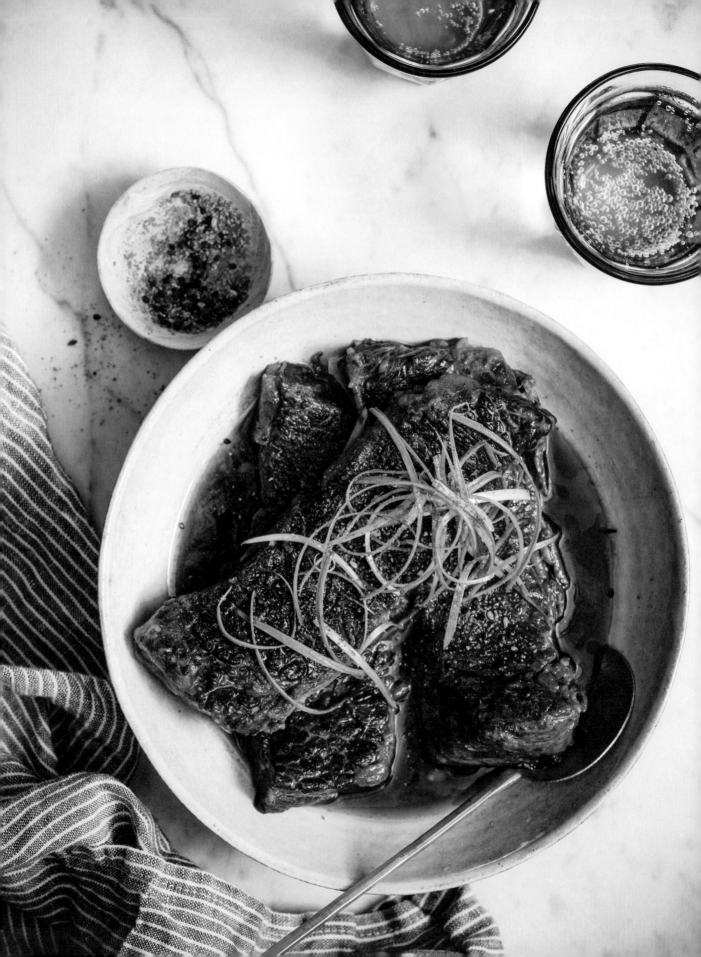

VARIATION: To make the short ribs in the oven, preheat the oven to 300°F. After seasoning with salt, sear the meat in a Dutch oven, then remove the meat to a plate and drain the oil. Add the soy sauce, sake, pineapple, sugar, garlic, ginger, and broth to the pot and stir gently to combine. Return the beef to the pot and top with the carrots and onions. Bring to a simmer over medium heat. Cover the pot and transfer to the oven. Roast until the meat is very tender and can be pulled apart with a fork, turning the meat once after 1½ hours, 3 to 4 hours total. Proceed with the recipe in Step 4.

QUICK TIP
Use 1½ cups Pineapple Teriyaki Glaze (page 186) instead of the soy sauce, sake, pineapple, sugar, garlic, and ginger.

MAKE AHEAD
This recipe is best prepared a day ahead. After returning the meat to the pot in Step 6, allow it to cool completely then refrigerate it overnight, which will make it easy to remove the fat that rises and hardens on top. The flavor will be even better on the second day.

NUTRITION INFORMATION (ABOUT 2½ OUNCES):
Calories: 358 | Added sugar: ¾ teaspoon or 3g | Carbohydrates: 12g | Sodium: 895mg | Saturated fat: 23% of calories or 9g | Fiber: 1g | Protein: 22g

SLOPPY JOES

Ingredients

1 tablespoon vegetable oil

1 cup chopped sweet onion

2 teaspoons chopped garlic

1½ teaspoons chili powder

1 teaspoon smoked paprika

½ teaspoon ground ginger

1 pound lean ground beef

½ teaspoon salt

Dash of freshly ground black pepper

1 can (6 ounces) low-sodium tomato paste

3 tablespoons Ketchup (page 190) or low-sugar ketchup

4 hamburger buns, warmed

SERVES 4

Sloppy Joes are making a comeback. Their homey flavor hits all the right comfort food notes, and they are super easy to prepare. But classic Sloppy Joes, especially the recipes that use canned sauces and ketchup, are high in added sugar. A typical Sloppy Joe recipe calls for about ½ cup ketchup plus added sugar, and the leading canned sauce clocks in at 1½ teaspoons per serving—plus there is sugar in the hamburger buns. To get that classic flavor without the sugar, this recipe uses smoked paprika and sweet onions along with homemade ketchup. There can be more than a teaspoon of sugar in each hamburger bun, so be sure to choose buns with no more than 4 grams of sugar per serving to go along with this meal. Serve with roasted sweet potato wedges.

1 Heat the oil in a skillet over medium-low heat. Add the onion, garlic, chili powder, paprika, and ginger and cook, stirring often and reducing the heat if necessary, until the onions are translucent and tender, 8 to 10 minutes.

2 Increase the heat to medium-high. Add the meat to the skillet with the onions, breaking it up a bit with a wooden spoon. Sprinkle with the salt and pepper. Let the meat brown, stirring, for 3 minutes. Stir in the tomato paste and ¾ cup (1 can) water. Scrape the bottom of the pan to loosen any browned bits, breaking up the meat some more. Add the ketchup and bring to a simmer. Reduce the heat to low and cook until the mixture is thick and saucy, about 10 minutes, stirring often. If needed, add more water, a tablespoon at a time, to reach desired consistency.

3 Divide the Sloppy Joe mixture among the buns and serve immediately.

QUICK TIP
Instead of homemade ketchup, use store-bought ketchup with less than 2 grams of sugar per tablespoon.

NUTRITION INFORMATION (1 SANDWICH):
Calories: 409 | Added sugar: ½ teaspoon or 2g | Carbohydrates: 35g | Sodium: 681mg | Saturated fat: 12% of calories or 5g | Fiber: 4g | Protein: 29g

MISO-GLAZED SALMON

OURS = 0 TEASPOONS
THEIRS = 3 TEASPOONS

Crushed pineapple and miso paste add sweet and salty flavor to this simple salmon dish. To maximize flavor, marinate the salmon overnight. Pair with sautéed greens and rice for a quick and easy weeknight dinner. You will have extra miso glaze left over—use it as a marinade for chicken, vegetables, or light fish.

1 Place the miso, pineapple, and sake in a blender. Blend until it forms a smooth glaze, about 1 minute.

2 Coat the salmon with 2 tablespoons of the glaze, cover tightly, and let sit in the refrigerator overnight or for up to 2 days. Reserve the remaining miso glaze for another use.

3 Place an oven rack 5 to 6 inches from the broiler. Preheat the oven to broil.

Line a rimmed baking sheet with aluminum foil and coat lightly with cooking spray.

4 Place the salmon skin side down on the prepared pan and remove any excess glaze or pineapple bits from the fish. Broil until just cooked through (be careful not to let it burn), 6 to 8 minutes. Let sit for a few minutes before serving.

☆ **MAKE AHEAD**
The miso glaze will keep in an airtight container in the refrigerator for up to 2 weeks.

Ingredients

½ cup white miso paste
¼ cup crushed pineapple, unsweetened or packed in juice, drained
¼ cup sake
4 skin-on salmon fillets (3 ounces each)
Nonstick cooking spray

SERVES 4

NUTRITION INFORMATION (1 SERVING):
Calories: 140 | Added sugar: 0 teaspoons or 0g | Carbohydrates: 2g | Sodium: 253mg | Saturated fat: 7% of calories or 1g | Fiber: 0g | Protein: 19g

POKE BOWLS

OURS = ¼ TEASPOON
THEIRS = 3¼ TEASPOONS

Ingredients

1 medium cucumber
(preferably seedless)

¾ teaspoon kosher salt

1 tablespoon unseasoned
rice vinegar

2 teaspoons canola oil,
for searing (optional)

1 pound sushi-grade raw
tuna or salmon, skin
removed (see headnote)

1 cup sushi rice or other
short-grain rice

2 tablespoons low-sodium
soy sauce

2 teaspoons toasted (dark)
sesame oil

1 teaspoon honey

2 green onions, trimmed
and thinly sliced

1½ teaspoons black
sesame seeds, plus
extra for garnish

2 tablespoons finely
shredded nori
(optional; see Notes)

OPTIONAL TOPPINGS

1 cup cooked, shelled
edamame

Cubed avocado

Cubed mango

Pickled ginger

Sliced jalapeño chiles

Wasabi paste or sriracha

Ponzu sauce (see Notes)

SERVES 4

A Hawaiian staple that's made its way to the mainland, poke is an increasingly popular quick-bites choice at fast-food restaurants. It's a simple chopped fish salad with myriad combinations of tasty toppings, but the raw fish is usually tossed with ultra-sweet sauces that are loaded with hidden added sugar. Our poke sauce is a simplified riff on the classic recipe, sweetened with a touch of honey. If you can't get sushi-grade fish, buy the best-quality tuna or salmon you can find and sear it—just cook it a couple hours ahead of time and chill it before serving. Instead of rice, you can also serve the poke and toppings over mixed greens.

1 Slice the cucumber crosswise into ½-inch pieces and place in a strainer over a bowl. Sprinkle the salt evenly over the cucumber and toss well to combine. Let sit for 15 minutes. Rinse under cold running water, then drain for another 5 minutes. Place in a serving bowl and toss with the vinegar.

2 If you are searing the fish, heat a nonstick skillet over medium-high heat until hot. Add the oil and heat until hot but not smoking, then place the fish flesh side down in the pan. Sear for 1 to 2 minutes per side, depending on how thick the fillet is. Transfer to a plate and let cool for 5 to 10 minutes, then cover loosely with plastic wrap and chill in the refrigerator for 1 to 2 hours.

3 About 30 minutes before you wish to eat, cook the rice according to the package directions. Set aside, covered, to keep warm.

4 Whisk together the soy sauce, sesame oil, and honey in a medium bowl.

Recipe continues

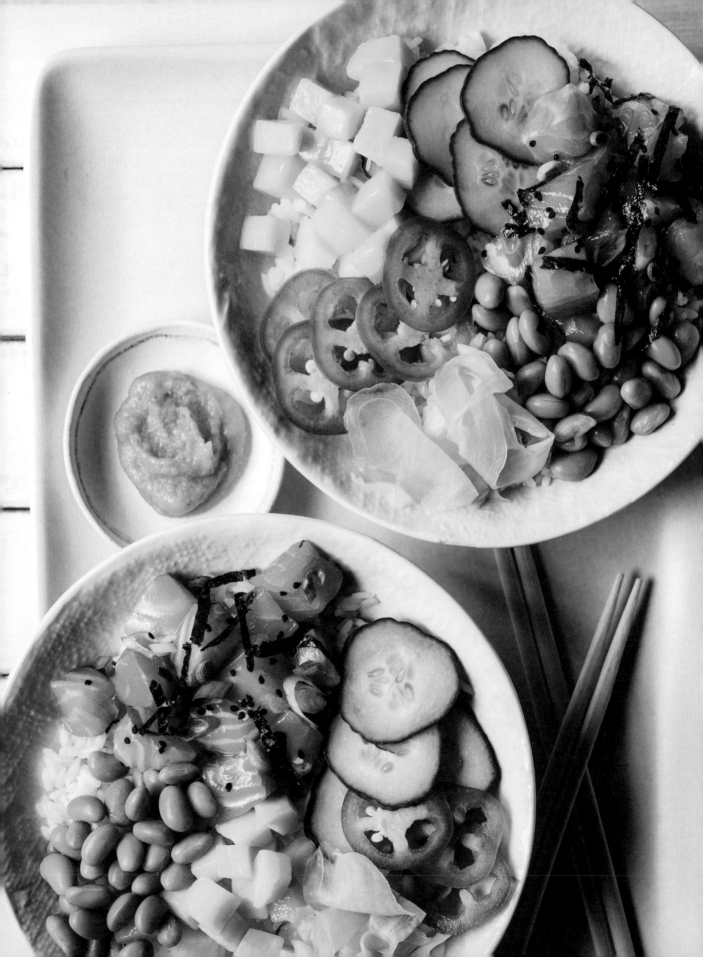

5 Cut the raw or seared fish into ½-inch cubes and place in a large bowl with the green onions, sesame seeds, and nori, if using. Add the sauce to the mixture and toss to combine.

6 To serve: Set out bowls of your toppings of choices, including the pickled cucumber, extra sesame seeds, and nori. Have everyone place a scoop of rice in their bowl and then top with some of the poke on one part of the bowl and the other toppings as they like.

NOTES: Nori is dried seaweed commonly used in Japanese cooking. Ponzu sauce is a classic Japanese citrus sauce (depending on the brand, it may contain a small amount of added sugar, so be sure to read the label). Both nori and ponzu can be found in most well-stocked grocery stores or online.

☺ **WHAT KIDS CAN DO**
Young chefs can help make the pickled cucumbers or set out the toppings.

NUTRITION INFORMATION (1 BOWL WITHOUT OPTIONAL TOPPINGS):
Calories: 343 | Added sugar: ¼ teaspoon or 1g | Carbohydrates: 43g | Sodium: 603mg | Saturated fat: 2% of calories or 1g | Fiber: 2g | Protein: 31g

SHRIMP PAD THAI

OURS = 1½ TEASPOONS
THEIRS = 3½ TEASPOONS

Many American versions of this Thai street food add ketchup, though the traditional dish is made with rock sugar, tamarind, and lots of fish sauce. This version uses less added sugar and sodium than usual and a bit of paprika for color. You can make it vegetarian by swapping extra tofu for the shrimp and using low-sodium soy sauce in place of the fish sauce.

1 Bring a large pot of water to a boil for the noodles. Cover the pot and reduce the heat to low.

2 Meanwhile, combine the sugar, vinegar, lime juice, soy sauce, fish sauce, paprika, and 2 tablespoons water in a small bowl, whisking to dissolve the sugar. Set aside.

3 When you are ready to start stir-frying (the next step), return the water to a full boil, remove from the heat, and add the noodles. Let soak until softened, 8 to 10 minutes, then drain.

4 Meanwhile, heat 1½ tablespoons of the oil in a wok or a large nonstick skillet over medium-high heat. Sauté the garlic until fragrant, about 10 seconds. Add the carrots and cabbage and stir-fry until wilted, 1 to 2 minutes. Add the shrimp and tofu and stir-fry until the shrimp just turns pink and the tofu is hot, about

2 minutes. Add the bean sprouts and green onions and stir-fry until just softened, about 1 minute more.

5 Add the noodles and sauce to the wok, making sure to scrape the bottom of the pan, and toss to coat. Reduce the heat and stir-fry until the noodles soak up the sauce, 2 to 4 minutes, adding a splash more water if it gets too dry.

6 Meanwhile, heat the remaining ½ tablespoon oil in a small nonstick pan over high heat. Add the eggs, reduce the heat, and scramble until just set, about 3 minutes.

7 Toss the eggs into the noodles and serve immediately, with the lime wedges alongside and the peanuts and red pepper flakes sprinkled on top.

☺ **WHAT KIDS CAN DO**
Kids can squeeze the limes.

Ingredients

2 tablespoons sugar

2 tablespoons unseasoned rice vinegar

1 tablespoon freshly squeezed lime juice, plus 1 lime, sliced into wedges

1 tablespoon low-sodium soy sauce

1 tablespoon fish sauce

1 teaspoon sweet paprika

7 ounces dried pad thai noodles or other narrow dried rice noodles

2 tablespoons roasted peanut oil or vegetable oil

1 teaspoon chopped garlic

1 cup carrot matchsticks

1 cup thinly sliced cabbage

8 ounces shelled and deveined large shrimp, halved lengthwise

7 to 8 ounces firm tofu, drained and cut into ½-inch strips

2 cups mung bean sprouts

2 green onions, trimmed, halved lengthwise, and cut into 1-inch lengths

2 large eggs, lightly beaten

½ cup chopped unsalted roasted peanuts, for garnish

Crushed red pepper flakes, for garnish

SERVES 4

NUTRITION INFORMATION (1 SERVING):
Calories: 590 | Added sugar: 1½ teaspoons or 6g | Carbohydrates: 63g | Sodium: 917mg | Saturated fat: 6% of calories or 4g | Fiber: 7g | Protein: 34g

PINEAPPLE TERIYAKI SALMON BURGERS
WITH SRIRACHA MAYO

OURS = ½ TEASPOON
THEIRS = 1¼ TEASPOONS

Ingredients

Nonstick cooking spray

2 green onions, trimmed and cut crosswise into 1-inch pieces

1 pound salmon fillet, skinned and deboned, cut into 1-inch chunks

¼ cup panko breadcrumbs

½ teaspoon kosher salt

1 large egg

3 tablespoons Pineapple Teriyaki Glaze (page 186)

6 tablespoons mayonnaise

1½ teaspoons sriracha

4 hamburger buns, lightly toasted

1 to 2 cups arugula

SERVES 4

The teriyaki flavor from the glaze is mild in these salmon burgers, but it gives them some juiciness. The sriracha mayo is a bit spicy, so you may want to let kids add it to taste. Keep the salmon as cold as possible before forming the patties to help them keep their shape. You can always fix their shape again on the pan.

1 Preheat the oven to 400°F. Line a rimmed baking sheet with aluminum foil and lightly coat with cooking spray.

2 Place the green onions in a food processor and pulse until chopped. Add the salmon and pulse a few times. Push down any large chunks and pulse a few more times, until roughly chopped. Add the breadcrumbs, salt, and egg and pulse until the mixture is just combined and starts to form into clumps while the salmon stays chunky. Don't overmix or it will turn the salmon into mush.

3 Gently form the salmon mixture into four patties about 4 inches in diameter and ¼ inch thick and place on the prepared baking sheet. Brush the tops liberally with 2 tablespoons of the teriyaki glaze. Bake until cooked on the bottom, 4 to 5 minutes, then flip and brush the tops with the remaining tablespoon of glaze. Return to the oven and bake until the patties are cooked through, 5 minutes more.

4 Combine the mayonnaise and sriracha in a small bowl. Spread the buns with the mayo, top with the salmon burgers and the arugula, and serve immediately.

NUTRITION INFORMATION (1 BURGER):
Calories: 418 | Added sugar: ½ teaspoon or 2g | Carbohydrates: 27g | Sodium: 775mg | Saturated fat: 9% of calories or 5g | Fiber: 1g | Protein: 31g

RAINBOW CHARD LASAGNA

OURS: 0 TEASPOONS
THEIRS: 1¼ TEASPOONS

This recipe is packed with vegetables, so when you need a healthy, one-pan dinner that feeds a crowd, you're covered. Tomato sauce is an unexpected source of added sugar, which is why many prepared lasagna dinners contain up to 2 teaspoons of added sugar per serving. Quick-Cook Tomato-Basil Sauce is an easy addition here, but if you're tight on time, you can use jarred sauce. Just be sure to use one that doesn't have added sugar in the ingredients list. You can also save time by swapping out the rainbow chard for frozen chopped spinach. Both are equally tasty and nutritious.

Ingredients

Nonstick cooking spray
Kosher salt
2 bunches rainbow chard, stems removed
Freshly ground black pepper
1 container (15 ounces) part-skim ricotta cheese
2 cups (8 ounces) shredded mozzarella
½ cup grated Parmesan cheese
5 cups Quick-Cook Tomato-Basil Sauce (page 188) or Slow-Cooker Tomato-Basil Sauce (page 189)
9 sheets oven-ready lasagna

SERVES 10

1 Preheat the oven to 375°F. Lightly coat a 13 × 9-inch baking dish with cooking spray.

2 Bring a large pot of salted water to a boil for the chard and set a strainer over a bowl near the stove. Blanch the chard leaves in batches until tender, 3 minutes. Remove with a slotted spoon or skimmer to the strainer. Let cool to the touch.

3 Move the strainer to the sink and squeeze the chard with your hands until very dry. Chop roughly and place it in a medium bowl. Toss with ¹⁄₁₆ teaspoon salt and pepper to taste.

4 Combine the ricotta, 1 cup of the mozzarella, and ¼ cup of the Parmesan in a medium bowl. Season with ¹⁄₁₆ teaspoon salt and pepper to taste.

5 Pour 1 cup of the sauce in the prepared baking dish and spread it in an even layer. Place 3 sheets of pasta on top in a single layer, leaving some space around them to allow them to expand when they cook. Add 1 cup of the sauce on top, spreading to cover the edges of the pasta. Sprinkle with half the rainbow chard, then dollop with half the ricotta cheese mixture. Spread or flatten the ricotta cheese gently with a large spoon (it will spread out more later).

6 Repeat the layers, starting with the sauce. Cover the final layer of pasta with the remaining 1 cup sauce, making sure to spread the sauce over the edges. Sprinkle the remaining 1 cup mozzarella and ¼ cup Parmesan on top.

7 Cover tightly with aluminum foil. Bake until the edges of the pasta are cooked through and the sauce is bubbly, about 35 minutes. Uncover and place under the broiler to brown, about 3 minutes.

Recipe continues

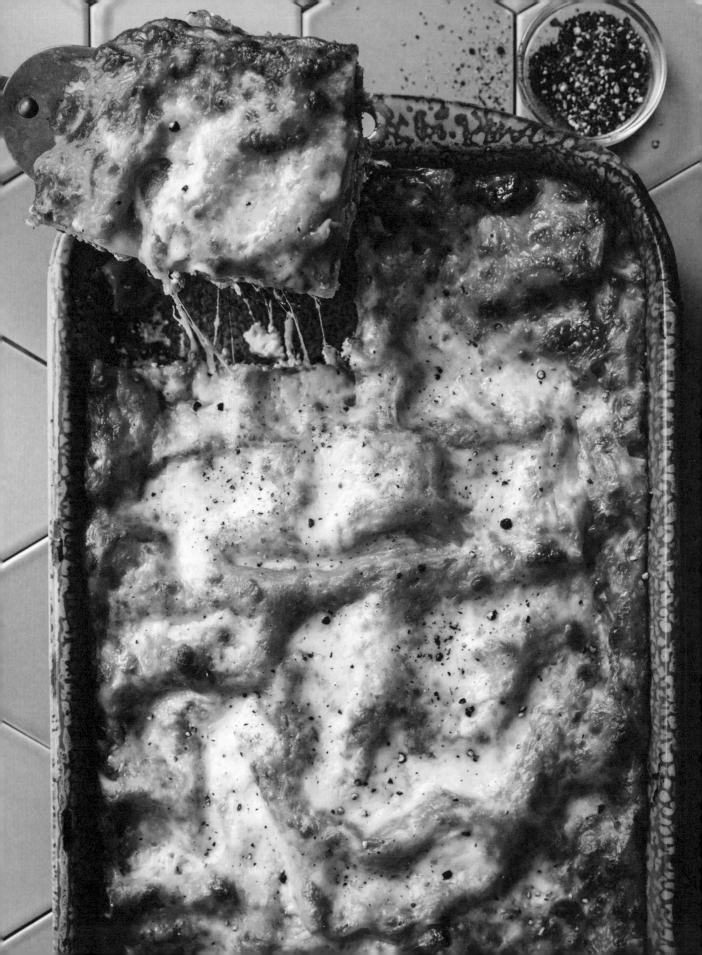

8 Remove from the oven and let rest, uncovered, for 15 to 20 minutes before cutting into 10 pieces and serving.

⚡ QUICK TIP

Use two jars (24 ounces each) no-added-sugar pasta sauce to save on cooking time (be sure to check the label for sugar or any of its derivative names). Instead of rainbow chard, you can use a 10-ounce package of frozen chopped spinach, thawed according to the package directions. Follow the same directions for squeezing the greens dry.

☺ WHAT KIDS CAN DO

Kids can tear the leaves from the rainbow chard. More experienced junior chefs can assemble the lasagna.

☆ MAKE AHEAD

You can assemble the lasagna ahead and store it, covered, in the refrigerator, then bake it the next day. Remove from the refrigerator and let sit at room temperature for 30 minutes while you preheat the oven. Make sure the sauce comes to a full boil in the oven. Leftover baked lasagna will keep, tightly wrapped in plastic wrap, in the freezer for up to 3 months. Thaw overnight in the refrigerator before reheating in the microwave.

NUTRITION INFORMATION (1 PIECE):
Calories: 285 | Added sugar: 0 teaspoons or 0g | Carbohydrates: 30g | Sodium: 825mg | Saturated fat: 17% of calories or 5g | Fiber: 6g | Protein: 16g

BBQ CHICKEN PIZZA

 OURS: ½ TEASPOON
THEIRS = 2 TEASPOONS

Ingredients

All-purpose flour,
  for dusting
1 recipe Overnight Pizza
  Dough (page 202)
  or 1 pound fresh pizza
  dough
2 teaspoons extra-virgin
  olive oil
½ cup BBQ Sauce
  (page 185)
1½ cups leftover shredded
  BBQ Chicken
  (page 96)
⅓ cup fresh corn kernels
3 ounces smoked
  mozzarella, sliced into
  thin strips, or grated
  smoked Gouda cheese
3 ounces shredded
  mozzarella cheese
1 green onion, trimmed
  and sliced
¼ cup chopped fresh
  cilantro (optional)
Crushed red pepper flakes,
  for garnish (optional)

SERVES 5

Inspired by a creation at a popular pizza chain, many versions of BBQ chicken pizza are loaded with sweet barbecue sauce and cheese. This one has tender pieces of chicken, a light coating of not-too-sweet sauce, and some smoked cheese for extra flavor. With the sweet corn and green onions, it's a delicious combination of flavors. Adults may want to add a sprinkle of red pepper flakes when it comes out of the oven to bring it all together.

1 Preheat the oven to 500°F.

2 Meanwhile, place the dough on a surface lightly dusted with flour, sprinkle the dough with flour, cover with a clean dish towel, and let sit at room temperature for 30 minutes.

3 Grease a rimmed baking sheet with the olive oil. Hold the dough in your hands and stretch it a bit in the form of a rectangle. Place the dough in the pan and use your fingers to stretch and pull it toward the corners of the pan so that it covers the pan evenly, taking care not to tear it (if it does, just patch the holes). The dough may not reach the corners, and that's fine, but make sure it's not too thick in the center.

4 Spread the BBQ sauce on the dough with a spoon, leaving a 1-inch border around the edges. Sprinkle the chicken and corn on top, then layer with the smoked cheese slices. Sprinkle with the shredded mozzarella to fill in the empty spots, then top with the green onion and the cilantro, if using.

5 Bake until the crust and cheese are browned and the sauce and cheese are bubbly, 11 to 13 minutes. Let cool slightly, then cut into 10 slices. Serve, sprinkled with the red pepper flakes, if using.

⚡ **QUICK TIP**
Use 1½ cups shredded rotisserie chicken (skin removed) if you don't have leftover BBQ Chicken on hand.

☺ **WHAT KIDS CAN DO**
Little chefs can add the toppings.

NUTRITION INFORMATION (2 SLICES):
Calories: 422 | Added sugar: ½ teaspoon or 2g | Carbohydrates: 48g |
Sodium: 654mg | Saturated fat: 13% of calories or 6g | Fiber 2g | Protein: 24g

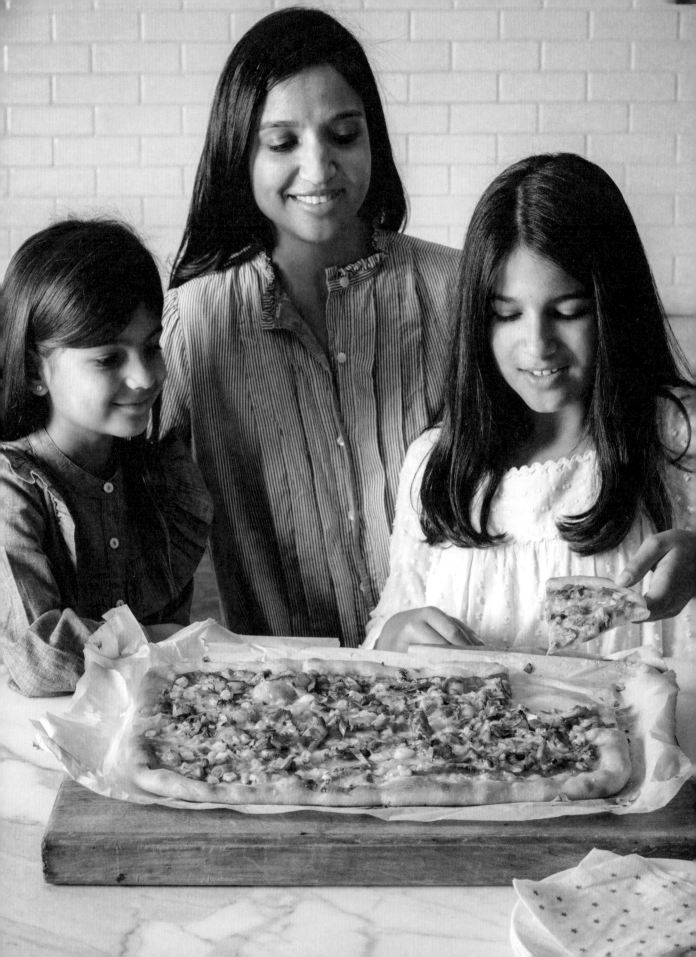

GRAM'S MEATBALLS AND SPAGHETTI

OURS = 0 TEASPOON*
THEIRS = 1½ TEASPOONS

Ingredients

FOR GRAM'S MEATBALLS
Nonstick cooking spray
12 ounces lean ground
    beef (90% lean)
8 ounces ground pork
2 large eggs
½ cup panko breadcrumbs
½ cup grated Parmesan
    cheese
¼ cup finely chopped flat-
    leaf (Italian) parsley
    (about ¼ bunch)
½ teaspoon salt
¼ teaspoon garlic powder
2 tablespoons extra-virgin
    olive oil

FOR THE SPAGHETTI
1 pound spaghetti
½ recipe (2½ cups) Quick-
    Cook Tomato-Basil
    Sauce (page 188) or
    Slow-Cooker Tomato
    Basil Sauce (page 189),
    warmed
Grated Parmesan cheese,
    for serving (optional)

SERVES 6

This modified version of Jennifer's Gram's original recipe is made simpler with oven baking, so you don't need to stand at the stove frying meatballs. A quick sauté in the pan gives the meatballs beautiful crispy edges, then you pop them in the oven to finish while you get the rest of the meal on the table.

1 Make the meatballs: Preheat the oven to 400°F. Lightly coat a rimmed baking sheet with cooking spray.

2 Using clean hands, mix together the beef, pork, eggs, breadcrumbs, Parmesan, parsley, salt, and garlic powder in a large bowl. Form into 12 meatballs, each about 2 inches in diameter.

3 Heat a large skillet over medium heat. Add 1 tablespoon of the oil and swirl to coat the pan. When hot, add half of the meatballs and cook, turning with tongs to brown most sides, about 4 minutes total. Remove to the prepared baking sheet. Repeat with the remaining oil and meatballs.

4 Bake the meatballs until cooked through and a thermometer inserted into the center reads 155°F to 160°F, about 15 minutes.

5 Make the spaghetti: Bring a large pot of salted water to a boil, add the spaghetti, and cook according to the package directions. Drain the pasta and return to the pot. Over low heat, toss the pasta with 2 cups of the sauce.

6 Spoon the spaghetti into warm pasta bowls, top each with 2 meatballs, and drizzle the meatballs with some of the remaining ½ cup sauce. Sprinkle with Parmesan, if you like, and serve immediately.

⭐ **MAKE AHEAD**
You can brown the meatballs 1 day ahead. Let cool, then refrigerate them in an airtight container. Finish in the oven the next day, adding an extra 5 to 10 minutes baking time. You can also freeze the cooked meatballs, tightly wrapped in plastic wrap, for 2 months. Unwrap and thaw the cooked meatballs on a plate in the refrigerator overnight. Bring to room temperature, about 30 minutes, then reheat in a 350°F oven until warmed through, 10 to 15 minutes.

NUTRITION INFORMATION (1 SERVING):
Calories: 676 | Added sugar: 0 teaspoons or 0g | Carbohydrates: 72g |
Sodium: 684mg | Saturated fat: 11% of calories or 8g | Fiber: 5g | Protein: 34g

*Negligible (there is a small amount of added sugar in the panko)

SPINACH-RICOTTA CALZONES

OURS = 0 TEASPOONS
THEIRS = ½ TEASPOON

This quick and easy variation on pizza is a crowd-pleasing comfort food. It's stuffed with spinach and ricotta, but you can feel free to mix and match using your favorite vegetables. Halved cherry tomatoes, sautéed mushrooms, or steamed chard (squeezed dry after cooling) all work well. The best part—our homemade tomato sauces eliminate the hidden sugars that often lurk in ready-made calzones.

1 Remove the dough from the refrigerator and cut into two equal portions. Form each into a ball and let sit at room temperature for at least 20 minutes.

2 Preheat the oven to 450°F. Grease a rimmed baking sheet with 1 tablespoon of the olive oil.

3 Sprinkle a work surface with flour and form each ball of dough into a 12-inch circle.

4 Combine the ricotta and egg in a medium bowl, then fold in the spinach, salt, and pepper.

5 Spread about ¼ cup sauce on half of each round of dough, leaving a ½-inch border.

6 Sprinkle half of the mozzarella on top of each and dot with spoonfuls of the ricotta mixture. Dollop the remaining ½ cup sauce on the ricotta. Layer the salami on top, if using. Fold over the top of the dough to cover the fillings and pinch to seal. Brush with the remaining 2 tablespoons olive oil.

7 Using a bench scraper or large offset spatula, carefully transfer the calzones to the prepared baking sheet. Bake until cooked through and golden brown, 22 to 25 minutes. Let cool for at least 5 minutes before slicing in half and serving. Be careful because they will be hot.

😊 WHAT KIDS CAN DO
Kids can sprinkle the cheese and salami, if using.

☆ MAKE AHEAD
Assemble the calzones, set on the greased pan, and cover the pan with plastic wrap. They will keep in the refrigerator for up to 24 hours. Remove from the refrigerator, unwrap, and let sit at room temperature for 30 minutes before baking as directed.

Ingredients

1 recipe Overnight Pizza Dough (page 202) or 1 pound fresh pizza dough

3 tablespoons extra-virgin olive oil

All-purpose flour, for dusting

1 cup part-skim ricotta cheese

1 large egg

10 ounces frozen chopped spinach, thawed and squeezed until very dry

¼ teaspoon salt

⅛ teaspoon freshly ground black pepper

1 cup Quick-Cook Tomato-Basil Sauce (page 188) or 5-Minute Marinara Dipping Sauce (page 104)

1 cup (4 ounces) shredded part-skim mozzarella cheese

8 slices dry salami (optional)

SERVES 4

NUTRITION INFORMATION (½ CALZONE):
Calories: 549 | Added sugar: 0 teaspoons or 0g | Carbohydrates: 60g | Sodium: 840mg | Saturated fat: 13% of calories or 8g | Fiber: 5g | Protein: 23g

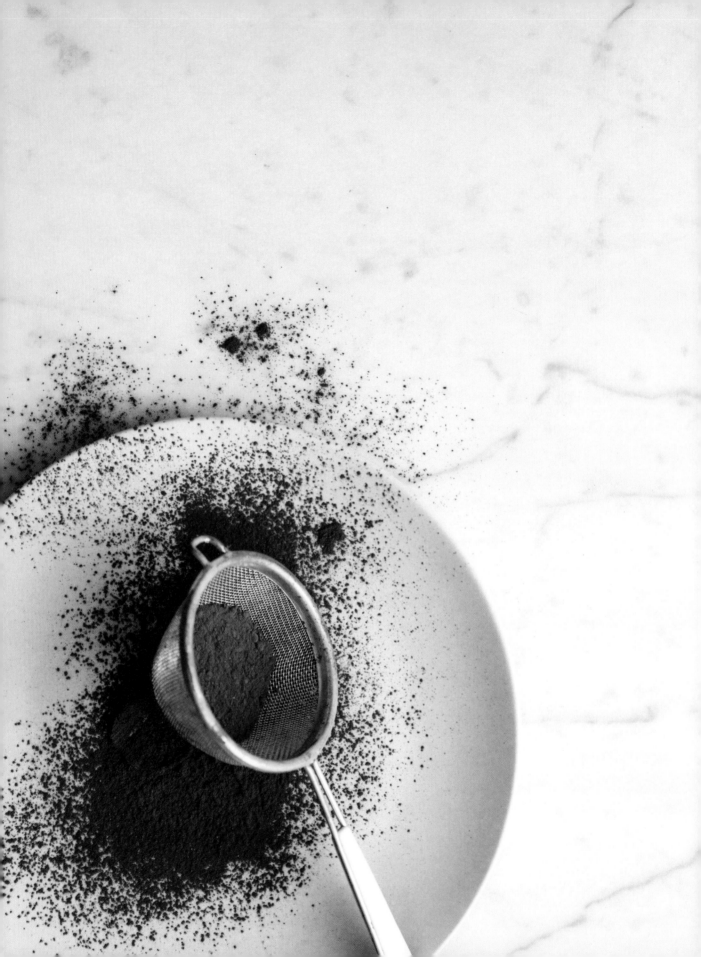

DESSERTS

Desserts represent about 20 percent of the added sugar we consume, so limiting them to special occasions and reducing the added sugar can make a big positive impact on your health. We took all our favorite family desserts—chewy chocolate chip cookies, decadent chocolate brownies, and sweet and salty caramel confections—and remastered them with no more than half the sugar. There are some desserts—like sorbets and meringues—that you won't find here because they rely on certain amounts of sugar for structure and taste. For those types of desserts, it's better to have the original as a once-in-a-while indulgence. But when you want to have a treat, the recipes here will allow you to enjoy many of your favorites with half the sugar and all of the flavor that you crave.

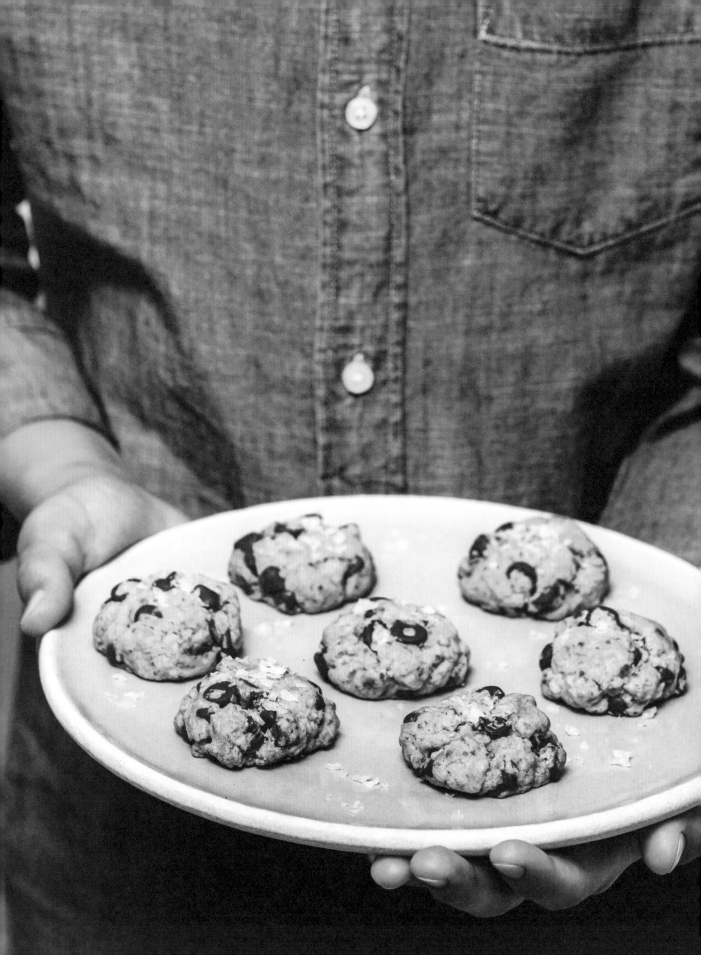

CHEWY CHOCOLATE CHIP COOKIES

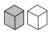 OURS = 1 TEASPOON
THEIRS = 2 TEASPOONS

You'd be hard pressed to find much of a difference between these chocolate chip cookies and tried-and-true ones, even though these have half the sugar of traditional cookies their size. Naturally sweet dates are pulverized into the flour and sub for the white sugar. Dark chocolate chips bring down the sugar level another notch. The lower baking temperature and baking soda help these lower-sugar cookies get crisp and golden brown around the edges. Expect a chewy cookie instead of a crispy one, with a little bit of chocolate in each bite.

1 Combine the flour and dates in a food processor fitted with a metal blade. Process until the dates are finely ground into the flour and the mixture looks like sand but is not clumpy, about 1 minute. Add the salt and baking soda and pulse until just combined. Set aside.

2 Mix together the melted butter and brown sugar in a stand mixer fitted with a paddle attachment (or using a handheld mixer) at medium speed until just combined, 1 minute.

3 Add the egg and egg yolks one at a time, mixing between additions. Add the vanilla and mix at medium speed until the mixture has a consistent color, another 1 to 2 minutes. Scrape down the side of the bowl.

4 With the mixer on low, working in three or four small batches, add the flour mixture until just combined. Stir in the chocolate chips with a silicone spatula,

making sure to gently fold the dough so that it's fully combined and there isn't any flour sitting at the bottom of the bowl. The dough will be a little soft at this point. Refrigerate it for 30 minutes.

5 Arrange a rack in the center of the oven. Preheat the oven to 325°F. Line two rimmed baking sheets with parchment paper.

6 Place rounded tablespoonfuls of dough on the prepared baking sheets, leaving 2 inches between cookies. Gently and slightly flatten the cookie dough rounds with the back of a spoon. This will help create a flatter and chewier cookie.

7 Sprinkle each cookie with a small pinch of sea salt. Bake, one sheet at a time, until the bottoms and edges are golden brown, 13 to 15 minutes. Let cool on the pan for 10 minutes, then transfer to wire racks to finish cooling completely. (If you put the cookies on a plate too early, they'll have soggy bottoms.)

Recipe continues

Ingredients

2 cups all-purpose flour

11 ounces Medjool dates, pitted (about 13 dates; see Note)

1 teaspoon salt

½ teaspoon baking soda

1 cup (2 sticks) unsalted butter, melted and cooled until just warm

⅓ cup packed light brown sugar

1 large egg plus 2 large egg yolks

2 teaspoons pure vanilla extract

10 ounces dark chocolate chips (about 1⅔ cups)

Flaky sea salt, for sprinkling

MAKES 48 COOKIES

NOTE: When making the date flour, do not overprocess the mixture. There may be a few flecks of date in the flour, and that's fine. If you process the date-flour mixture too long, it will turn into dough—as a result of the dates breaking down too much—and will be difficult to combine with the butter-sugar mixture.

☺ **WHAT KIDS CAN DO**
Kids can stir in the chocolate chips and portion out the cookies.

☆ **MAKE AHEAD**
To freeze, portion out the dough on a prepared baking sheet, wrap tightly with plastic wrap, then cover with aluminum foil and freeze for at least 6 hours. Once frozen, remove the portioned dough from the baking sheet, place in a resealable plastic bag or airtight container, and store in the freezer for up to 1 month. When you're ready to bake, thaw completely, then follow directions from Step 6.

Because of the lower sugar content, these cookies won't keep as long as traditional cookies. They are best enjoyed the day they are made but will keep in an airtight container at room temperature for up to 3 days. They may get a little soft by the second day because of the water content in the dates. The cookies can be firmed up by heating them in a 375°F oven for 5 to 10 minutes before serving.

NUTRITION INFORMATION (1 COOKIE):
Calories: 112 | Added sugar: 1 teaspoon or 4g | Carbohydrates: 14g | Sodium: 68mg | Saturated fat: 29% of calories or 4g | Fiber: 1g | Protein: 1g

CREATING THE PERFECT COOKIE

It took three chefs more than twenty-five tries to get to what our tasters thought was the perfect low-sugar version of the iconic chocolate chip cookie. We started by using date puree to sweeten the cookies. The flavor was excellent, but the high water content of the puree resulted in cake-like cookies with a damp texture. We knew we had to eliminate water, so we tried pulverizing the dates into the flour to add sweetness without too much moisture. Better, but not perfect.

Texture was still an issue, so we added two egg yolks. Egg whites produce dry and often cakey cookies and require more sugar to neutralize their effect. Yolks added richness and provided a crispy exterior and a chewier interior. We also took out the baking powder, since the acid in it tends to make baked goods puffier (or in this case, cakier). We kept a small amount of baking soda as a neutralizer, which allowed the cookies to brown more in the oven without rising.

We also experimented with the type of sugar. Our initial batches used granulated sugar, but we eventually opted for light brown sugar not only because it helped deliver that quintessential chocolate chip cookie flavor but also because it helped with texture. Brown sugar absorbs moisture after baking, making cookies chewy even after they cool. Finally, we added an extra teaspoon of pure vanilla extract, because when the vanilla flavor is up front rather than just a background note, it seems to scream classic chocolate chip cookie. The result: a low-sugar cookie that is nearly indistinguishable from that classic golden brown, rich, buttery, slightly chewy chocolate chip cookie that you're craving.

PEANUT BUTTER COOKIES

OURS: ¾ TEASPOON
THEIRS: 1¾ TEASPOONS

Creamy peanut butter and dates come together to sweeten this irresistible peanut butter cookie with less than half the sugar of a typical recipe. Like our Chewy Chocolate Chip Cookies (page 131), these cookies required lots of testing to get that classic peanut butter cookie flavor and texture. Melted butter works best here so that you can work the dough less, making the cookies more tender. Extra vanilla extract and a touch of salt bring out the rich peanut butter flavor and round out the sweetness. We also added two extra egg yolks, so that the outside of the cookie has a nice crisp texture, but the interior is soft and chewy.

1 Combine the flour and dates in a food processor fitted with a metal blade. Process until the dates are finely ground into the flour and the mixture looks like sand but is not clumpy, about 1 minute. Add the salt, baking powder, and baking soda and pulse until just combined. Set aside.

2 Mix together the melted butter, peanut butter, and brown sugar in a stand mixer fitted with a paddle attachment (or use a handheld mixer) at medium speed until just combined, 1 minute.

3 Add the egg and egg yolks one at a time, mixing between additions. Add the vanilla and mix at medium speed until the mixture has a consistent color, another 1 to 2 minutes. Scrape down the side of the bowl.

4 With the mixer on low, working in three or four small batches, add the flour mixture until just combined. The dough will be a little soft at this point. Refrigerate it for 30 minutes.

5 Arrange a rack in the center of the oven. Preheat the oven to 325°F. Line two rimmed baking sheets with parchment paper.

6 Place rounded tablespoonfuls of dough on the prepared baking sheets, leaving 2 inches between cookies. Gently flatten each cookie in a crisscross pattern with a fork. Sprinkle with the chopped peanuts, if using.

7 Bake, one sheet at a time, until the cookies are slightly browned, 11 to 13 minutes. Do not overbake or the cookies will crumble. Let cool on the pan for 10 minutes, then transfer to wire racks to finish cooling completely. (If you put the cookies on a plate too early, they'll have soggy bottoms.)

Ingredients

2 cups all-purpose flour
8 ounces Medjool dates, pitted (about 10 dates)
1½ teaspoons salt
1 teaspoon baking powder
¾ teaspoon baking soda
1 cup (2 sticks) unsalted butter, melted and slightly cooled
⅔ cup unsweetened, unsalted peanut butter
½ cup packed light brown sugar
1 large egg plus 2 large egg yolks
2 teaspoons pure vanilla extract
¼ cup finely chopped peanuts (optional)

MAKES 40 COOKIES

Recipe continues

☺ WHAT KIDS CAN DO

Kids can measure the ingredients and portion out the cookies.

☆ MAKE AHEAD

To freeze, portion out the dough on a prepared baking sheet, wrap tightly with plastic wrap, then cover with aluminum foil and freeze for at least 6 hours. Once frozen, remove the portioned dough from the baking sheet, place in a resealable plastic bag or airtight container, and store in the freezer for up to 1 month.

When you're ready to bake, thaw completely, then follow directions from Step 6.

Because of the lower sugar content, these cookies won't keep as long as traditional cookies. They are best enjoyed the day they are made but will keep in an airtight container at room temperature for up to 3 days. They may get a little soft by the second day because of the water content in the dates. The cookies can be firmed up by heating them in a 375°F oven for 5 to 10 minutes before serving.

NUTRITION INFORMATION (1 COOKIE):
Calories: 122 | Added sugar: ¾ teaspoon or 3g | Carbohydrates: 13g | Sodium: 115mg | Saturated fat: 25% of calories or 3g | Fiber: 1g | Protein: 2g

BLONDIES
WITH WHITE CHOCOLATE AND ALMONDS

OURS = 1¾ TEASPOONS
THEIRS = 4½ TO 6 TEASPOONS

The vanilla version of a classic brownie, blondies are a delicious treat. Dates add a note of caramel in this recipe and sub for a significant portion of the brown sugar that is typically used. There are just enough white chocolate and dark chocolate chips to ensure that you get a little bit of chocolate with each bite. These clock in at about 70 percent less added sugar than a typical blondie.

1 Preheat the oven to 325°F. Line a 13 × 9-inch baking dish with parchment paper, leaving 2 inches of overhang on each side, and coat with cooking spray.

2 Combine the flour and dates in a food processor fitted with a metal blade. Process until the dates are finely ground into the flour and the mixture looks like sand but is not clumpy, about 1 minute. Add the salt and baking soda and pulse until just combined. Set aside.

3 Mix together the melted butter and brown sugar in a stand mixer fitted with a paddle attachment (or using a handheld mixer) at medium speed until just combined, 1 minute.

4 Add the eggs and egg yolks one at a time, mixing between additions. Add the vanilla and mix at medium speed until the

mixture has a consistent color, 1 to 2 minutes more. Scrape down the side of the bowl.

5 With the mixer on low, working in three or four small batches, add the flour mixture until just combined. Stir in ½ cup of the white chocolate chips, the dark chocolate chips, and the almonds with a silicone spatula, making sure to gently fold the batter so that it's fully combined and there isn't any flour sitting at the bottom of the mixer bowl.

6 Transfer the batter to the prepared baking dish, spread into an even layer, and sprinkle with the remaining 2 tablespoons white chocolate chips. Bake until a toothpick inserted into the center comes out with a few moist crumbs, about 25 minutes.

7 Let the blondies cool completely. Cut into 24 bars.

Ingredients

Nonstick cooking spray
1¾ cups all-purpose flour
8 ounces Medjool dates, pitted (about 10 dates)
1½ teaspoons salt
½ teaspoon baking soda
1 cup (2 sticks) unsalted butter, melted and cooled until just warm
⅓ cup packed light brown sugar
2 large eggs plus 2 large egg yolks
1½ teaspoons pure vanilla extract
½ cup plus 2 tablespoons white chocolate chips (3¾ ounces)
½ cup dark chocolate chips (3 ounces)
¾ cup slivered almonds, toasted

MAKES 24 BARS

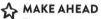 **MAKE AHEAD**
The bars will keep, tightly wrapped in plastic wrap, in the refrigerator for up to 2 days or in the freezer for up to 1 month.

NUTRITION INFORMATION (1 BAR):
Calories: 217 | Added sugar: 1¾ teaspoons or 7g | Carbohydrates: 23g | Sodium: 185 mg | Saturated fat: 28% of calories or 7g | Fiber: 2g | Protein: 3g

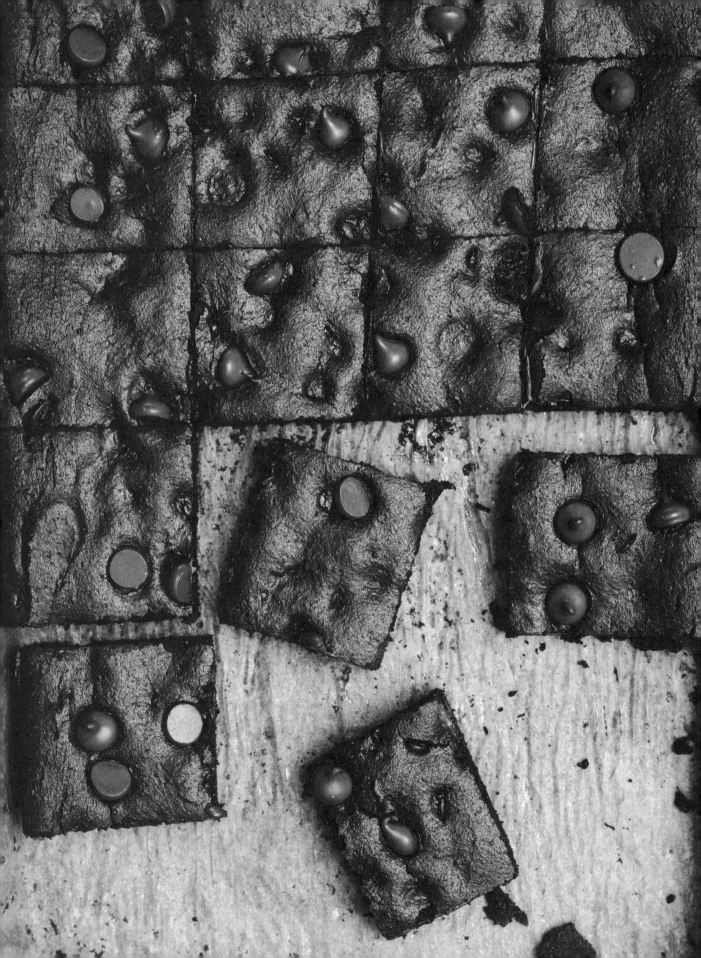

DOUBLE CHOCOLATE BROWNIES

OURS: 1½ TEASPOONS
THEIRS: 4½ TEASPOONS

Our rich, fudgy brownies hit the mark with less than half the sugar of a boxed brownie mix. The secret ingredients are ones that none of our tasters could guess: sweet potatoes and almond butter. Sweet potatoes give these brownies a natural sweetness, while almond butter adds a creamy, rich texture—plus they're studded with chocolate chips. They don't need flour, so they're great for gluten-free families. If you use canned sweet potato puree, the whole recipe comes together in less than 10 minutes in the food processor, so you can satisfy chocolate cravings quickly.

Ingredients

Nonstick cooking spray
½ pound sweet potatoes, peeled, cubed, and boiled until fork-tender
½ cup unsweetened almond butter
½ cup coconut oil or unsalted butter (1 stick), melted
1 large egg plus 1 large egg yolk
¼ cup maple syrup
2 teaspoons pure vanilla extract
¾ cup unsweetened natural cocoa powder
½ teaspoon salt
½ teaspoon baking soda
1 cup plus 2 tablespoons semisweet chocolate chips (6¾ ounces)

MAKES 24 BROWNIES

1 Preheat the oven to 350°F. Line a 13 × 9-inch baking dish with parchment paper, leaving 2 inches of overhang on each side, and coat with cooking spray.

2 Combine the sweet potatoes, almond butter, coconut oil, egg, and egg yolk in a food processor. Process until very smooth, making sure no chunks of sweet potato remain, about 1 minute.

3 Scrape down the side of the bowl and add the maple syrup and vanilla. Process until combined, about 30 seconds.

4 Add the cocoa powder, salt, and baking soda and process until all the dry ingredients are incorporated, about 1 minute more. Fold in 1 cup of the chocolate chips.

5 Pour the batter into the prepared pan, spread it into an even layer, and sprinkle with the remaining 2 tablespoons chocolate chips. Bake until the top is set and a toothpick inserted into the center comes out with a few moist crumbs, 27 to 30 minutes. Let the brownies cool slightly. Cut into 24 bars.

⚡ **QUICK TIP**
You can substitute 1 cup canned sweet potato puree for the fresh sweet potato.

☺ **WHAT KIDS CAN DO**
Little chefs can measure the ingredients and sprinkle the chocolate chips.

☆ **MAKE AHEAD**
The brownies can be stored in an airtight container at room temperature for up to 3 days.

NUTRITION INFORMATION (1 BROWNIE):
Calories: 136 | Added sugar: 1½ teaspoons or 6g | Carbohydrates: 12g | Sodium: 97mg | Saturated fat: 30% of calories or 5g | Fiber: 2g | Protein: 3g

SALTED CARAMEL CHOCOLATE CHEESECAKE BARS

▦▦▦▢ OURS = 1¾ TEASPOONS
THEIRS = 4 TEASPOONS

Ingredients

Nonstick cooking spray

FOR THE CRUST
8 ounces Medjool dates,
    pitted (about 10 dates)
6 ounces (about 1½ cups)
    shelled raw walnuts
½ teaspoon salt

FOR THE FILLING
1 package (8 ounces)
    cream cheese,
    at room temperature
¾ cup nonfat plain Greek
    yogurt
¼ cup maple syrup
2 teaspoons freshly
    squeezed lemon juice
1 teaspoon pure vanilla
    extract
1 teaspoon salt
2 large eggs
½ cup Salted Maple-
    Date Caramel Sauce
    (page 200) plus
    3 tablespoons for
    the topping

FOR THE TOPPINGS
⅓ cup semisweet chocolate
    chips (2 ounces)
⅓ cup toasted peanuts
Dash of flaky sea salt

MAKES 16 BARS

Salted caramel, rich chocolate, and toasted peanuts come together in this indulgent cheesecake bar that's reminiscent of a classic, oh-so-satisfying candy bar. With a decadent recipe like this, we had to push the limits on how to swap ingredients to drop the added sugar. We started with the crust because this cheesecake bar needed a strong foundation. We tried both a graham cracker crust and a nut and date crust. Although the graham cracker crust gave these bars a traditional cheesecake feel, the date and nut crust allowed us to drop the added sugar, boost healthy ingredients, and add some depth of flavor that the other crust just couldn't achieve. We swapped out half of the cream cheese for low-fat Greek yogurt, which helps keep this recipe within saturated fat targets for a dessert. The combination mimics the creaminess of traditional cheesecake. It does add a little tartness, which is mellowed with the richness of the chocolate and peanuts. For the delicious topping, we used Salted Maple-Date Caramel Sauce, roasted peanuts, and a drizzle of chocolate. These bars are definitely a special-occasion treat, but you can feel good knowing they are still well within your daily limit of added sugar!

1 Line an 8 × 8-inch baking pan with parchment paper, leaving about 2 inches of overhang on each side. Coat lightly with cooking spray.

2 Make the crust: Combine the dates, walnuts, and salt in a food processor fitted with a metal blade and process until well blended and no pieces of dates remain.

3 Use your fingers to press the mixture into the prepared pan. Then, using a flat surface like the bottom of a glass or an offset spatula, press down until the mixture is firmly packed. Freeze until ready to use, at least 30 minutes.

4 Preheat the oven to 375°F.

5 Make the filling: Beat the cream cheese in the bowl of a stand mixer fitted with a paddle attachment at medium speed until smooth, about 1 minute. Add the yogurt and beat until combined, scraping down the side of the bowl as needed. Add the maple syrup, lemon juice, vanilla, salt, and eggs and continue beating until smooth and no clumps of cream cheese remain, about 1 minute more.

6 Remove the crust from the freezer. Pour the filling on top of the frozen crust and spread into an even layer. Dollop the ½ cup of caramel sauce in small spoonfuls over the entire surface, then use a toothpick to swirl it into the cheesecake.

7 Bake until the edges are set and the center jiggles only slightly, about 35 minutes. Check the cheesecake at 25 minutes. If it's beginning to brown too much, tent it with foil.

8 Remove the cheesecake from the oven and let cool slightly, about 20 minutes. Put in the freezer until just chilled, 15 to 20 minutes.

9 Meanwhile, place the chocolate chips in a medium microwave-safe bowl. Microwave, stirring at 30-second intervals, until the chocolate is just melted, about 1½ minutes total.

10 Sprinkle the peanuts over the surface of the chilled cheesecake, pressing them down slightly so they adhere. Dollop the remaining 3 tablespoons caramel sauce over the surface. Using the edge of an offset spatula, drizzle the melted chocolate over the top. Sprinkle with the flaky salt.

11 Place in the freezer until the chocolate sets, about 5 minutes. To slice, warm a knife under hot water and dry fully to ensure that all water is removed. Cut the cheesecake into 16 squares. Serve cold.

☺ WHAT KIDS CAN DO
Place the melted chocolate in a resealable plastic bag, cut off a small corner of the bag, and let kids pipe on the chocolate drizzle!

☆ MAKE AHEAD
These bars can be stored, unsliced and tightly wrapped in plastic wrap, in the refrigerator for 1 week or in the freezer for up to 1 month.

NUTRITION INFORMATION (1 BAR):
Calories: 255 | Added sugar: 1¾ teaspoons or 7g | Carbohydrates: 26g | Sodium: 293mg | Saturated fat: 17% of calories or 5g | Fiber: 2g | Protein: 6g

SALTED NUT BUTTER CRISPY RICE TREATS

OURS = 1 TEASPOON
THEIRS = 2 TEASPOONS

Ingredients

Nonstick cooking spray
4 cups brown rice cereal
6 tablespoons (¾ stick)
    unsalted butter
¼ cup honey
¾ cup unsweetened
    peanut or almond
    butter
2 teaspoons pure vanilla
    extract
Dash of flaky sea salt,
    for topping

MAKES 16 BARS

Retooling the classic chewy rice cereal treats took a lot of trial and error. We tried to make them with a homemade marshmallow fluff, but ultimately this honey and nut butter combination yielded the best result with the least amount of sugar. Browned butter adds an extra layer of depth and deliciousness. Although not exactly like the original, these salty and sweet treats are addictive with their crunchy-gooey combination. This recipe works equally well with almond butter or peanut butter, so feel free to use your favorite spread. Because this recipe doesn't have much sugar, the bars will crumble at room temperature—they are best served cold.

1 Line an 8 × 8-inch baking pan with parchment paper, leaving about 2 inches of overhang on each side. Lightly coat the parchment paper with cooking spray.

2 Place the rice cereal in a large bowl; set aside.

3 Brown the butter in a medium saucepan over medium heat until darkened in color and fragrant, about 4 minutes. Add the honey and whisk to combine. Bring to a vigorous simmer and cook until frothy, about 1 minute. Add the nut butter and vanilla and stir until the nut butter is fully melted and incorporated into the honey butter. Remove the mixture from the heat and let cool slightly.

4 Pour the warm butter mixture over the rice cereal and stir to combine. Press the mixture into the prepared pan, using the bottom edge of an offset spatula or the bottom of a glass to firmly compress it in the pan. Sprinkle with the sea salt.

5 Freeze until firm, 25 minutes. Cut into 16 squares and serve cold.

☺ **WHAT KIDS CAN DO**
Little chefs can press the mixture into the pan.

☆ **MAKE AHEAD**
The treats will keep, tightly wrapped in plastic wrap, in the refrigerator for 2 to 3 days or in the freezer for up to 1 month.

NUTRITION INFORMATION (1 BAR):
Calories: 162 | Added sugar: 1 teaspoon or 4g | Carbohydrates: 14g | Sodium: 12mg | Saturated fat: 21% of calories or 4g | Fiber: 2g | Protein: 4g

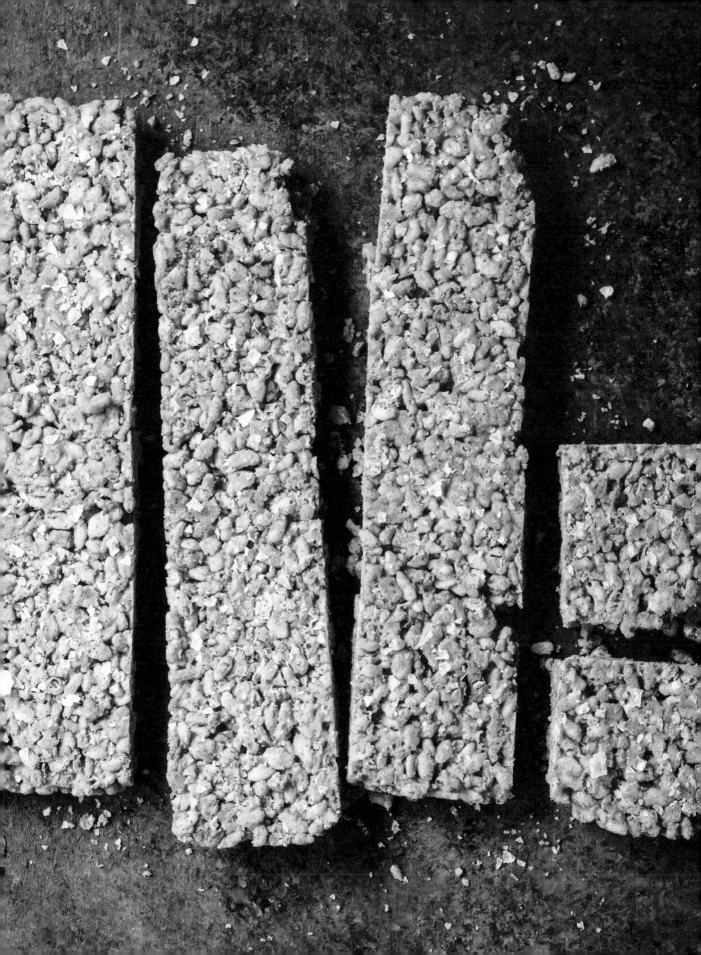

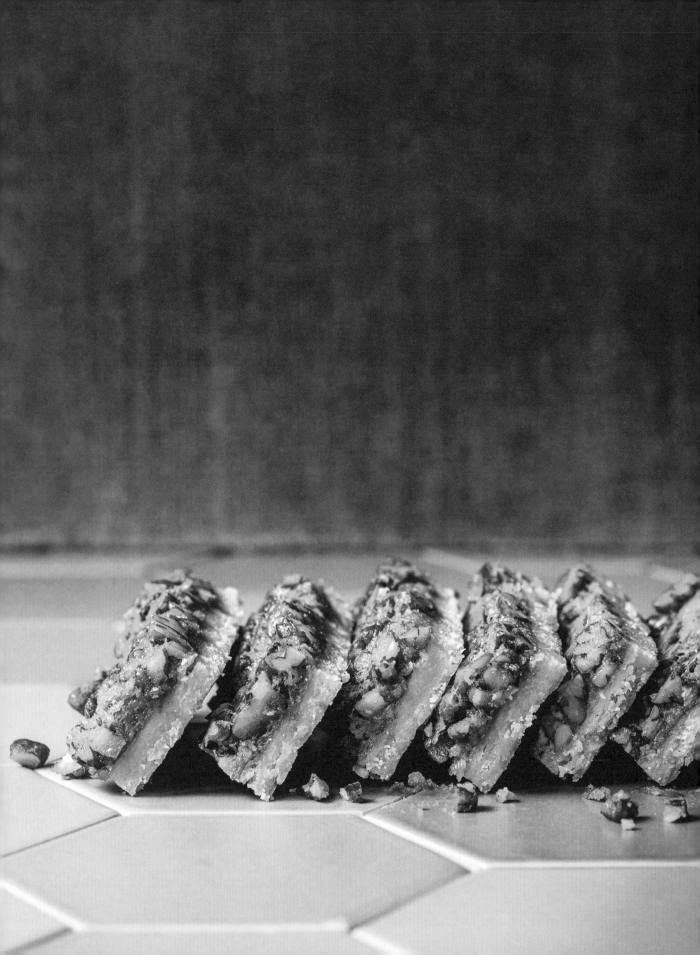

PECAN PIE BARS

OURS: 2 TEASPOONS
THEIRS: 4 TEASPOONS

Pecan pie is an all-American classic, but it's typically loaded with more sugar than pecans. Remastering the recipe was a challenge. We tried several variations with many different types of sugar, including honey and maple syrup. Ultimately, we found that a combination of light corn syrup and brown sugar was right here in order to achieve that classic gooey center with half the sugar of a typical pecan pie bar recipe. Toasting the pecans before baking is key because it adds depth of flavor.

1 Preheat the oven to 350°F. Line an 8 × 8-inch baking pan with parchment paper, leaving about 2 inches of overhang on each side.

2 Make the crust: Place the flour in a medium bowl.

3 Place the butter, brown sugar, salt, and 3 tablespoons water in a small microwave-safe bowl or measuring cup. Microwave, stirring at 30-second intervals, until melted and hot, 1 to 2 minutes. Stir, then immediately pour the butter mixture into the flour. Stir until a dough forms and the edges pull away from the bowl. Let the dough cool briefly.

4 When the dough is just cool enough to handle, use your fingers to spread it in an even layer in the prepared baking pan. Bake the crust until lightly golden brown on the edges, 20 to 22 minutes.

5 Meanwhile, make the filling: Spread the pecans on a rimmed baking sheet and toast until golden brown with a nutty aroma, about 5 minutes, watching closely to prevent burning. Let cool briefly.

6 Whisk together the corn syrup, brown sugar, butter, vanilla, and salt in a medium bowl. Beat in the eggs, then stir in the pecans.

7 When the crust comes out of the oven, spread the filling evenly on top and return to the oven. Bake until the filling is set and browned and the crust is firm all the way through, 30 minutes more. Let cool in the pan for at least 15 minutes. Cut into 20 bars. The bars are best served fully cooled.

Ingredients

FOR THE CRUST

1 cup all-purpose flour
7 tablespoons unsalted butter, chopped
1 tablespoon packed light brown sugar
½ teaspoon salt

FOR THE FILLING

1¼ cups chopped pecans
¼ cup plus 2 tablespoons light corn syrup
¼ cup packed light brown sugar
4 tablespoons (½ stick) unsalted butter, melted
2 teaspoons pure vanilla extract
¼ teaspoon salt
2 large eggs

MAKES 20 BARS

⭐ **MAKE AHEAD**
The bars will keep, tightly wrapped in plastic wrap, at room temperature for up to 3 days or in the freezer for up to 1 month.

NUTRITION INFORMATION (1 BAR):
Calories: 166 | Added sugar: 2 teaspoons or 8g | Carbohydrates: 14g | Sodium: 100mg | Saturated fat: 25% of calories or 5g | Fiber: 1g | Protein: 2g

BLUEBERRY PIE ⬡

Ingredients

1 prepared (9-inch) pie crust, homemade (page 203) or store-bought

7 cups blueberries (about 36 ounces)

3 tablespoons cornstarch

2 teaspoons finely grated lemon zest

1½ teaspoons ground cinnamon

½ teaspoon salt

1 teaspoon pure vanilla extract

1 large egg

Maple-Vanilla Whipped Cream (page 199), for serving (optional)

SERVES 8

Juicy, sweet blueberries are the stars in this classic summertime pie. No added sugar is required! A touch of cinnamon complements the berries, and lemon zest adds brightness. It's delicious with a dollop of Maple-Vanilla Whipped Cream for a treat. The dough cutouts are optional, but if you wish to make them, save the scraps from the crust (or use an extra crust), roll them out to an ⅛-inch thickness, and cut out shapes with cookie cutters.

1 Preheat the oven to 400°F.

2 Place 4 cups of the blueberries in a saucepan set over medium heat. Cook, smashing occasionally with a wooden spoon or potato masher, until mostly broken down and reduced, 15 to 20 minutes. Let cool completely.

3 Meanwhile, combine the remaining 3 cups blueberries with the cornstarch, lemon zest, cinnamon, salt, and vanilla in a large bowl. Add the cooled cooked blueberries and stir to combine. Transfer the mixture to the pie crust.

4 Whisk together the egg and 1 tablespoon water in a small bowl to make an egg wash. Brush the egg wash on the edges of the pie crust (and the dough cutouts, if using).

5 Place the pie on a rimmed baking sheet (if using the dough cutouts, arrange them on top of the filling) and bake for 25 minutes. Reduce the oven temperature to 350°F and continue to bake until the crust is golden brown and most of the blueberry liquid has evaporated, 15 minutes more. Remove from the oven and cool completely, 2 hours. (Because this pie has no added sugar, it takes more time to fully set.) Slice and serve with the whipped cream, if you like.

⚡ **QUICK TIP**
Use a store-bought pastry crust to cut down on time. Choose one with no added sugar if possible.

NUTRITION INFORMATION (1 SLICE):
Calories: 256 | Added sugar: 0 teaspoons or 0g | Carbohydrates: 34g | Sodium: 303mg | Saturated fat: 26% of calories or 7g | Fiber: 4g | Protein: 4g

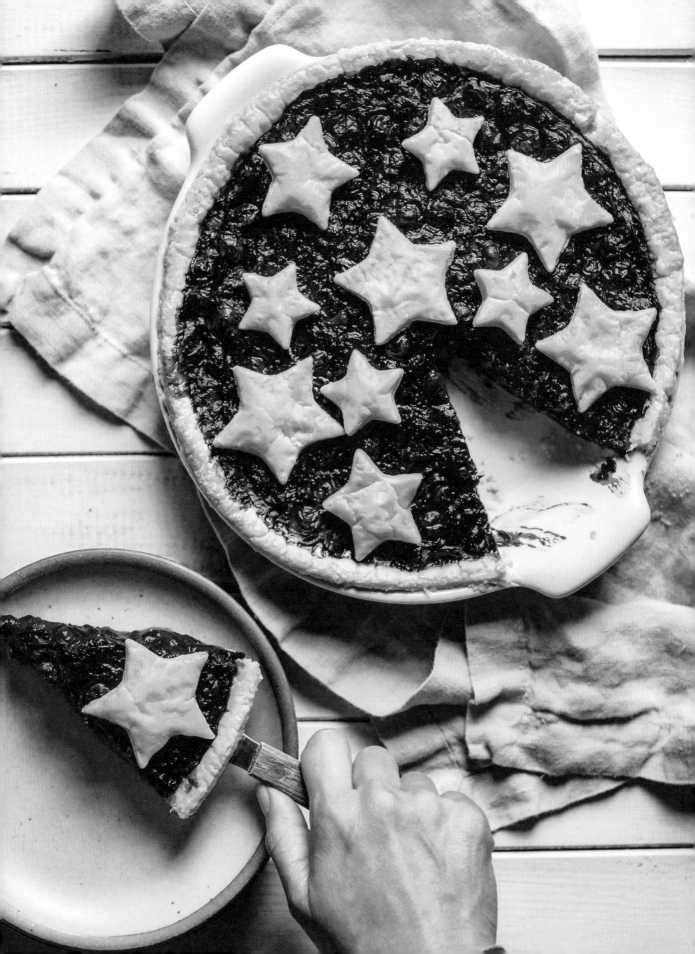

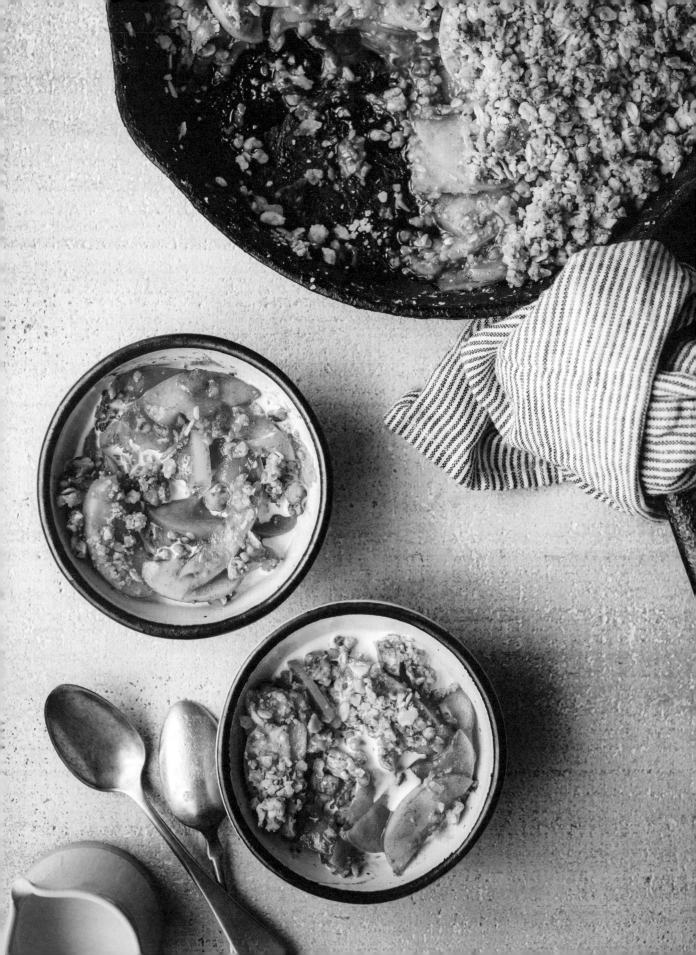

APPLE CRISP

OURS: 1½ TEASPOONS
THEIRS: 4 TO 5 TEASPOONS

This comforting apple crisp is packed with all the delicious flavors of a traditional apple pie but is much easier to make. Apples play the starring role in this dish, and if you use ripe, sweet ones like Braeburns, you don't need to add much sugar. To reduce the sugar in the topping, we loaded it up with toasted pecans, oats, and spices.

1 Preheat the oven to 350°F. Coat a 13 × 9-inch baking dish or a large cast-iron skillet with cooking spray.

2 Make the filling: Place the apples in a large mixing bowl. Combine the sugar, cornstarch, cinnamon, and salt in a small bowl and sprinkle over the apples. Drizzle the lemon juice and butter over the apples and toss to coat evenly.

3 Make the topping: Place the flour, pecans, oats, sugar, cinnamon, nutmeg, and salt in a food processor and pulse until the nuts and oats are finely chopped, about 30 seconds. Add the butter and pulse until clumpy, about 30 seconds more.

4 Spread the apple mixture evenly in the prepared baking dish, then sprinkle with the topping.

5 Bake until the topping is golden brown and the apples are tender when pierced with a knife, about 1 hour.

6 Serve warm, with a drizzle of heavy cream, if you like.

VARIATION: This recipe can also be made with peaches. Simply double the cornstarch that you mix into the fruit and bake until the fruit is tender, about 45 minutes.

☺ **WHAT KIDS CAN DO**
Little ones will delight in sprinkling the topping over the apples. More advanced junior chefs can peel and slice the apples.

☆ **MAKE AHEAD**
You can assemble the crisp several hours in advance. Cover and refrigerate until you're ready to bake. The baked crisp will keep, tightly wrapped in plastic wrap, in the refrigerator for up to 3 days.

NUTRITION INFORMATION (1 SERVING):
Calories: 254 | Added sugar: 1½ teaspoons or 6g | Carbohydrates: 35g | Sodium: 178mg | Saturated fat: 19% of calories or 5g | Fiber: 5g | Protein: 2g

Ingredients

Nonstick cooking spray

FOR THE FILLING
3 pounds sweet apples (like Braeburns, not Granny Smiths), peeled, cored, and sliced into ¼-inch wedges
1 tablespoon sugar
1 tablespoon cornstarch
2 teaspoons ground cinnamon
½ teaspoon salt
2 tablespoons freshly squeezed lemon juice
1 tablespoon unsalted butter, melted

FOR THE TOPPING
½ cup all-purpose flour
½ cup chopped pecans
½ cup old-fashioned (rolled) oats
¼ cup sugar
½ teaspoon ground cinnamon
¼ teaspoon ground nutmeg or ground allspice
¼ teaspoon salt
6 tablespoons (¾ stick) unsalted butter, melted
Heavy cream or Maple-Vanilla Whipped Cream (page 199), for serving (optional)

SERVES 10

CARAMELIZED PUMPKIN PIE

OURS = 2 TEASPOONS
THEIRS = 4¾ TEASPOONS

Ingredients

23 ounces canned
pumpkin puree
(about 2¾ cups; see
Note, page 35)

⅓ cup maple syrup

¼ cup low-fat milk or
almond milk

3¾ teaspoons pumpkin pie
spice (see Note)

2½ teaspoons pure vanilla
extract

½ teaspoon salt

4 large eggs plus 1 large
egg yolk, gently
whisked

1 prepared (8-inch) pie
crust, blind baked and
cooled completely
(see page 203)

Maple-Vanilla Whipped
Cream (page 199),
for serving (optional)

SERVES 8

Caramelizing pumpkin puree with maple syrup brings out the natural sweetness of the winter squash in this irresistible pie. That simple trick also concentrates the sweetness of the maple syrup, resulting in a decadent dessert that uses less than half the sugar of a traditional pumpkin pie recipe. Serve it up with a dollop of Maple-Vanilla Whipped Cream, if you choose.

1 Preheat the oven to 350°F. Combine the pumpkin puree with the maple syrup in a medium saucepan over medium heat. Cook, stirring frequently, until slightly darkened and caramelized, 5 to 7 minutes. Transfer to a large bowl and let cool completely.

2 Add the milk, pumpkin pie spice, vanilla, salt, and egg mixture and stir until well combined. Pour into the pie crust and smooth into an even layer. Bake until the top is slightly browned and the filling is set throughout, about 50 minutes.

3 Let the pie cool completely before slicing. Serve with the Maple-Vanilla Whipped Cream, if you like.

NOTE: If you don't have pumpkin pie spice on hand, you can create a substitute by combining 2 teaspoons ground cinnamon, 1 teaspoon ground ginger, ½ teaspoon ground nutmeg, and ¼ teaspoon ground cloves or ground allspice.

⚡ QUICK TIP
Use a store-bought pastry crust to cut down on time. Choose one with no added sugar if possible. Blind bake it as directed on page 203.

NUTRITION INFORMATION (1 SLICE):
Calories: 273 | Added sugar: 2 teaspoons or 8g | Carbohydrates: 29g |
Sodium: 338mg | Saturated fat: 28% of calories or 8g | Fiber: 3g | Protein: 6g

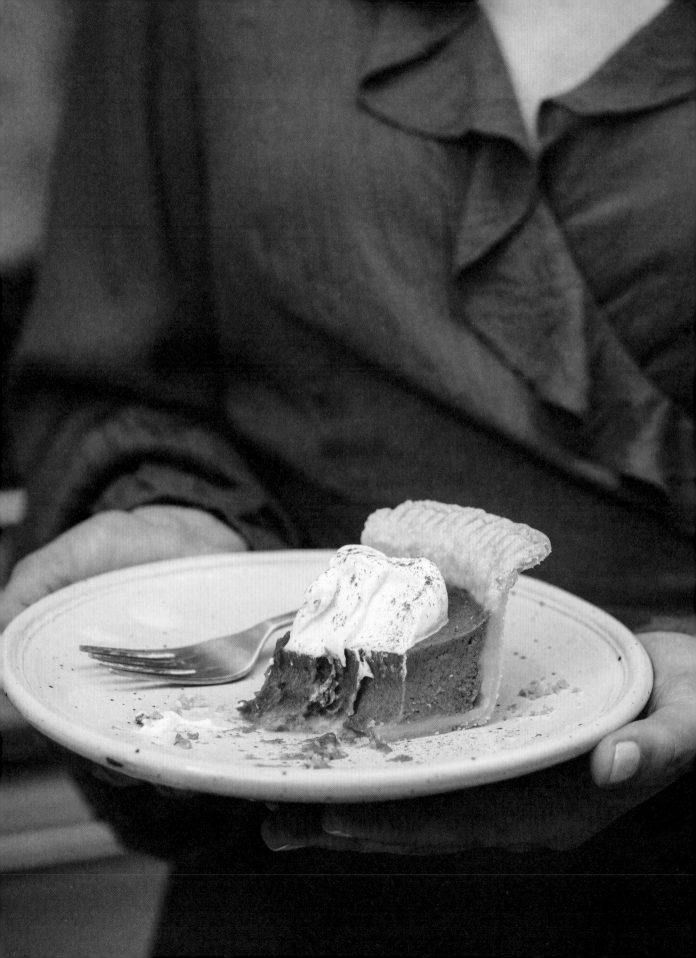

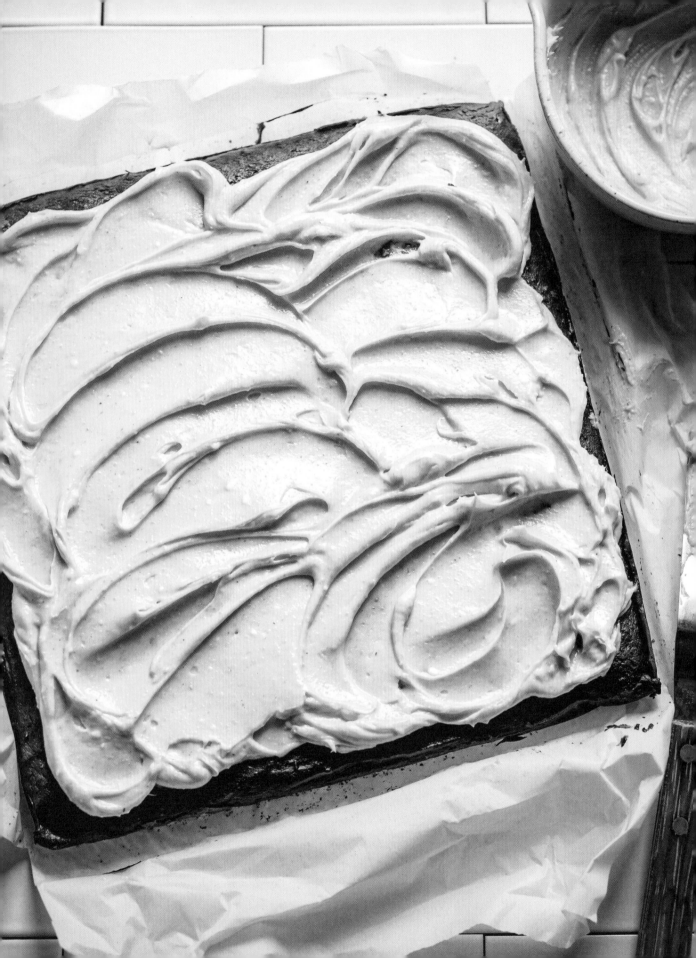

CHOCOLATE AND PEANUT BUTTER SNACK CAKE

OURS = 2¼ TEASPOONS
THEIRS = 7¼ TEASPOONS

We adore this decadent chocolate–peanut butter snack cake. It was a happy mistake that we stumbled on when trying to create a low-sugar brownie. The cake gets its richness from sweet dates combined with chocolate, cocoa powder, and vanilla. Creamy peanut butter in the frosting balances out this delicious bite. The flavor is intense!

1 Preheat the oven to 350°F. Line an 8 × 8-inch baking pan with parchment paper, leaving about 2 inches of overhang on each side. Coat lightly with cooking spray.

2 Place the dates in a medium bowl. Cover the dates with the hot water. Set aside until the dates are softened, about 10 minutes. Drain the dates, reserving ½ cup of the soaking liquid. Combine the dates and the reserved soaking liquid in a food processor fitted with a metal blade. Process until smooth, about 1 minute. Set aside.

3 Combine the butter and chocolate chips in a large heatproof bowl, set over a saucepan filled with 1 inch of simmering water, making sure the bottom of the bowl doesn't touch the water. Stir until melted. Remove from the heat and let cool slightly. Whisk in the sugar, vanilla, and eggs. Add the date puree and stir until combined. Add the flour, cocoa powder, salt, and baking powder and stir until combined.

4 Transfer the batter to the prepared pan, spread in an even layer, and bake until the top is set and a toothpick inserted into the center comes out clean, 15 to 20 minutes. Let the cake cool completely.

Recipe continues

Ingredients

FOR THE CAKE
Nonstick cooking spray
7 ounces Medjool dates, pitted (about 8 dates)
2 cups hot water
½ cup (1 stick) unsalted butter
5 ounces semisweet chocolate chips (about ¾ cup)
¼ cup sugar
2 teaspoons pure vanilla extract
2 large eggs
½ cup all-purpose flour
½ cup plus 2 tablespoons unsweetened natural cocoa powder
½ teaspoon salt
½ teaspoon baking powder

FOR THE PEANUT BUTTER FROSTING
½ cup (1 stick) unsalted butter, at room temperature
½ cup unsweetened peanut butter
1 tablespoon sugar
1 teaspoon pure vanilla extract
½ teaspoon salt

SERVES 16

5 Meanwhile, make the frosting: Beat the butter on medium speed in the bowl of a stand mixer fitted with a paddle attachment until smooth, about 2 minutes. Add the peanut butter and continue to beat until fully combined, about 1 minute, scraping down the side of the bowl as needed. Add the sugar, vanilla, and salt and mix until just combined.

6 Spread the frosting on the completely cooled cake and cut into 16 squares.

☺ **WHAT KIDS CAN DO**
Kids can spread the frosting (and lick the spatula).

☆ **MAKE AHEAD**
The cake will keep, tightly wrapped in plastic wrap, in the refrigerator for up to 1 week or in the freezer for 1 month.

NUTRITION INFORMATION (1 PIECE):
Calories: 276 | Added sugar: 2¼ teaspoons or 9g | Carbohydrates: 26g | Sodium: 197mg | Saturated fat: 32% of calories or 10g | Fiber: 3g | Protein: 5g

RED VELVET CUPCAKES
WITH CREAM CHEESE FROSTING

OURS: 3½ TEASPOONS
THEIRS: 8½ TEASPOONS

These remastered red velvet cupcakes are sweetened with applesauce to reduce added sugar. They get their crave-worthy, delicate crumb thanks to the addition of sour cream. Beet juice naturally adds a soft red hue, though the color won't be as bright as a typical red velvet cake made with commercial food dyes. The cream cheese frosting is sweet and creamy with just a bit of tang, perfect for topping these irresistible little cakes.

1 Preheat the oven to 350°F. Line a standard muffin pan with 12 paper liners.

2 Combine the flour, cocoa powder, baking soda, and salt in a medium bowl. Combine the applesauce and sour cream in a small bowl.

3 Beat the sugar and butter on medium-high speed in the bowl of a stand mixer fitted with a paddle attachment until light and fluffy, about 3 minutes. Add the eggs and vanilla and beat to combine. Add the flour mixture, alternating with the applesauce mixture, ending with the flour mixture, and beat until just combined. Add the beet juice and vinegar and beat until the batter is a consistent color.

4 Divide the batter evenly among the paper liners and bake until a toothpick inserted into the center of each cupcake comes out clean, 14 to 18 minutes (avoid overbaking, which will lead to discoloration). Let cool in the pan for 10 minutes, then remove from the pan and transfer to a wire rack to cool completely before frosting.

NOTE: Beet juice is available at natural foods supermarkets. If you'd prefer to make your food coloring from scratch, grate 2 large, raw red beets on the smallest holes of a box grater, then gather up the grated beets in a cheesecloth bundle. Squeeze and twist the bundle to press the beet juice into a bowl. The beets will stain, so be sure to wear rubber gloves.

Ingredients

1 cup all-purpose flour

2 tablespoons unsweetened natural cocoa powder

1¼ teaspoons baking soda

1 teaspoon salt

½ cup unsweetened applesauce

¼ cup sour cream

½ cup sugar

4 tablespoons (½ stick) unsalted butter, at room temperature

2 large eggs

1 tablespoon pure vanilla extract

⅓ cup beet juice (see Note)

2 teaspoons white vinegar

1 recipe Cream Cheese Frosting (page 154)

MAKES 12 CUPCAKES

NUTRITION INFORMATION (1 CUPCAKE WITH FROSTING):
Calories: 294 | Added sugar: 3½ teaspoons or 14g | Carbohydrates: 25g | Sodium: 406mg | Saturated fat: 36% of calories or 12g | Fiber: 1g | Protein: 4g

Cream Cheese Frosting

OURS: 1¼ TEASPOONS
THEIRS: 4¾ TEASPOONS

Ingredients

4 tablespoons (½ stick) unsalted butter, at room temperature

8 ounces cream cheese, chilled and cut into 1-inch pieces

5 tablespoons sugar

1 teaspoon pure vanilla extract

MAKES ENOUGH TO FROST 12 CUPCAKES

This sweet and creamy frosting gets a little bit of tang from cream cheese and is perfect paired with Red Velvet Cupcakes (page 153). It clocks in at nearly 75 percent less added sugar than packaged frosting, plus it's much more flavorful.

Beat the butter on medium speed in the bowl of a stand mixer fitted with a paddle attachment. With the mixer running, add the cream cheese, 1 piece at a time, until combined. Add the sugar and vanilla and beat until combined, scraping down the side of the bowl as needed.

☆ **MAKE AHEAD**
The frosting can be made a day ahead. It will keep in an airtight container in the refrigerator. Let it come to room temperature before using.

NUTRITION INFORMATION (PER CUPCAKE):
Calories: 155 | Added sugar: 1¼ teaspoons or 5g | Carbohydrates: 6g | Sodium: 61mg | Saturated fat: 50% of calories or 9g | Fiber: 0g | Protein: 1g

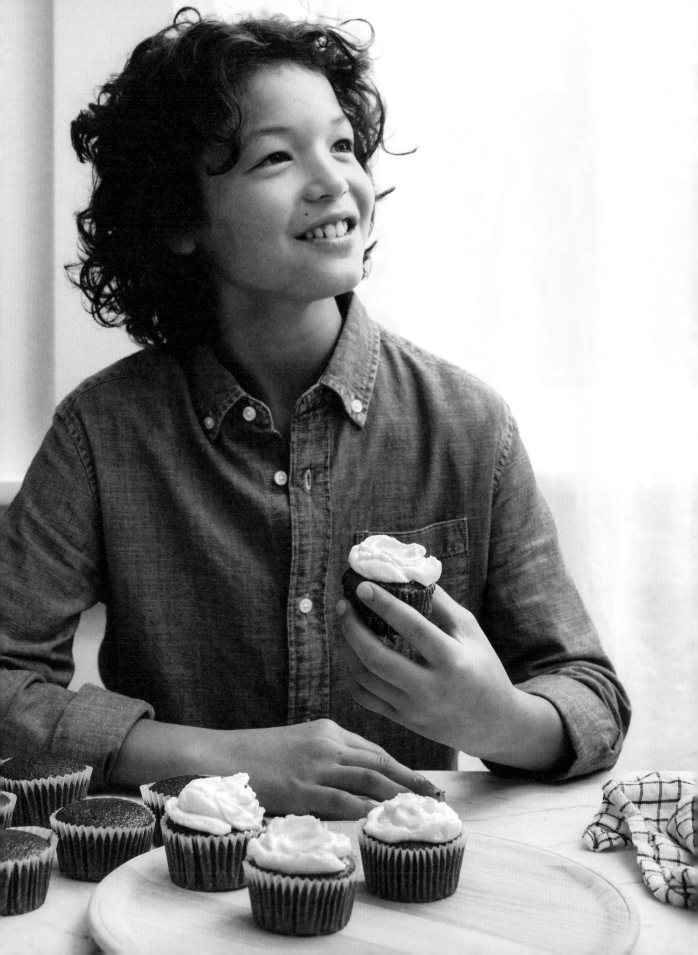

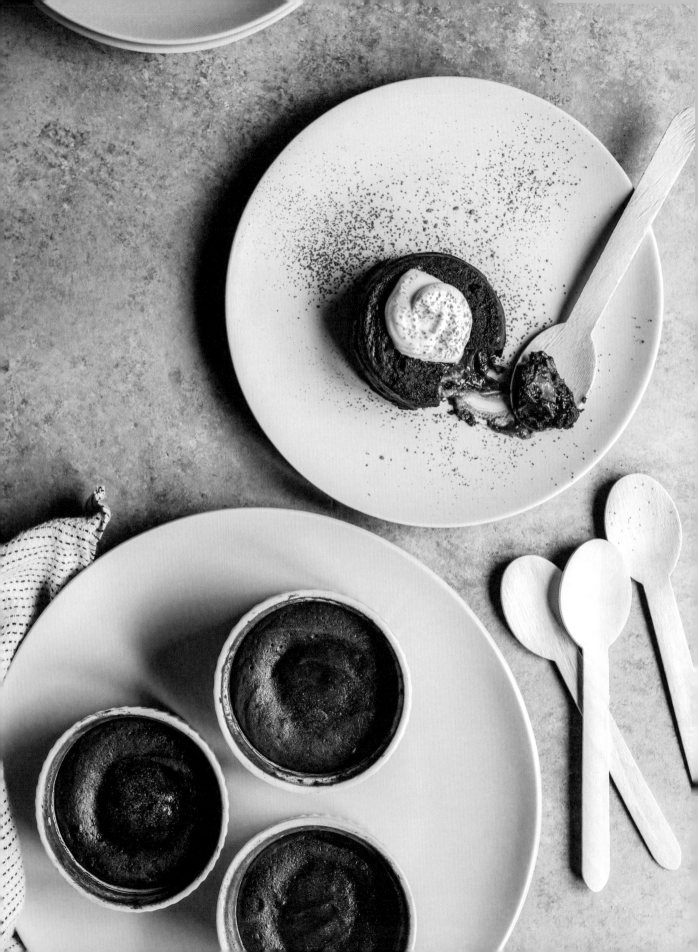

SALTED MAPLE-DATE CARAMEL MOLTEN CHOCOLATE CAKES

OURS = 5 TEASPOONS
THEIRS = 10¼ TEASPOONS

When you're craving a decadent treat, these easy-to-make molten chocolate cakes are the recipe to reach for. Typical versions of these popular lava cakes clock in at more than 10 teaspoons of added sugar per serving. Salted Maple-Date Caramel Sauce substitutes for the chocolate filling here, giving these cakes plenty of natural sweetness and an irresistible gooey center. These little gems are indulgent, but when the occasion calls for something extra special, they deliver.

Ingredients

Nonstick cooking spray

¼ cup unsweetened natural cocoa powder, plus extra for dusting

½ cup (1 stick) unsalted butter, cut into 8 equal pieces

4 ounces dark chocolate, chopped (about ⅔ cup)

¼ cup sugar

1 teaspoon pure vanilla extract

Dash of salt

3 large eggs

6 tablespoons Salted Maple-Date Caramel Sauce (page 200), chilled

¾ cup Maple-Vanilla Whipped cream (page 199), for serving

MAKES 6 INDIVIDUAL CAKES

1 Preheat the oven to 425°F. Coat the inside of six small (3-ounce) ramekins with cooking spray, lightly dust with cocoa powder, and place on a rimmed baking sheet.

2 Combine the butter and chocolate in a large heatproof bowl, set over a saucepan filled with 1-inch simmering water, making sure the bottom of the bowl doesn't touch the water. Stir until melted. Remove from the heat and let cool slightly.

3 Add the sugar, ¼ cup cocoa powder, the vanilla, salt, and eggs to the melted chocolate mixture and whisk to combine.

4 Divide half of the batter evenly among the ramekins. Carefully drop 1 tablespoon of the caramel sauce into the center of each ramekin, then top evenly with the remaining batter, making sure the sauce is fully covered with batter.

5 Bake until the sides are firm and centers are soft and look almost baked through, about 10 minutes. Let cool slightly. Using a kitchen towel to hold the ramekins, place a serving plate on top of each ramekin and invert the molten cake onto the plate, gently shaking the ramekin so that the cake comes out. Serve with the whipped cream and a dusting of the cocoa powder.

☺ WHAT KIDS CAN DO
Kids can dollop on the whipped cream and dust the cakes with cocoa powder.

☆ MAKE AHEAD
The cakes can be assembled the day before, covered, and stored in the refrigerator until you're ready to bake.

NUTRITION INFORMATION (1 CAKE WITH 2 TABLESPOONS WHIPPED CREAM):
Calories: 418 | Added sugar: 5 teaspoons or 20g | Carbohydrates: 32g | Sodium: 80mg | Saturated fat: 39% of calories or 18g | Fiber: 3g | Protein: 6g

DOUBLE CHOCOLATE LAYER CAKE
WITH WHIPPED CHOCOLATE FROSTING

OURS: 3¾ TEASPOONS
THEIRS: 10 TO 12 TEASPOONS

Ingredients

Nonstick cooking spray
1½ cups all-purpose flour
½ cup unsweetened
　natural cocoa powder
1½ teaspoons baking
　powder
1½ teaspoons salt
1 teaspoon baking soda
½ cup (1 stick) unsalted
　butter, at room
　temperature
⅓ cup sugar
2 large eggs
1 tablespoon pure vanilla
　extract
¾ cup whole milk
1 cup freshly brewed
　coffee, cooled slightly
2 teaspoons white vinegar
Whipped Chocolate
　Frosting (page 160)
Flaky sea salt, for garnish
　(optional)

SERVES 12

Rich and ultra chocolaty layers of chocolate cake are paired with whipped chocolate frosting for a decadent treat. Coffee adds a hint of robust flavor while also enhancing the rich chocolate flavor of unsweetened cocoa powder. It's the secret ingredient that pulls it all together. The cake layers are not as thick as those of a typical layer cake, but they are intense! When paired with a fluffy whipped chocolate frosting, this cake is beautifully balanced. It's perfect for your most special celebrations.

1 Preheat the oven to 350°F. Coat two 8-inch round cake pans with cooking spray. Line each pan with a round of parchment paper and coat the paper with cooking spray.

2 Combine the flour, cocoa powder, baking powder, salt, and baking soda in a medium bowl; set aside.

3 Beat the butter and sugar on medium speed in the bowl of a stand mixer fitted with a paddle attachment until light and fluffy, about 3 minutes. Add the eggs one at a time, beating after each addition. Add the vanilla, increase the speed to medium-high, and beat for 30 seconds.

4 Add the flour mixture in three additions, alternating with the milk, and beat on medium speed until just combined. With the mixer on low speed, slowly pour in the warm coffee. Once it is mostly incorporated, add the vinegar, increase the speed to medium-high, and beat for 30 seconds, scraping the bowl as needed.

5 Divide the batter evenly between the prepared cake pans and bake until a toothpick inserted into the center of each cake comes out clean, about 30 minutes. Let the layers cool in the pans for 10 minutes, then remove from the pans and transfer them to a wire rack to cool completely.

6 Set one cake layer on a stand and frost the top with about a third of the frosting. Top with the second cake layer and frost the

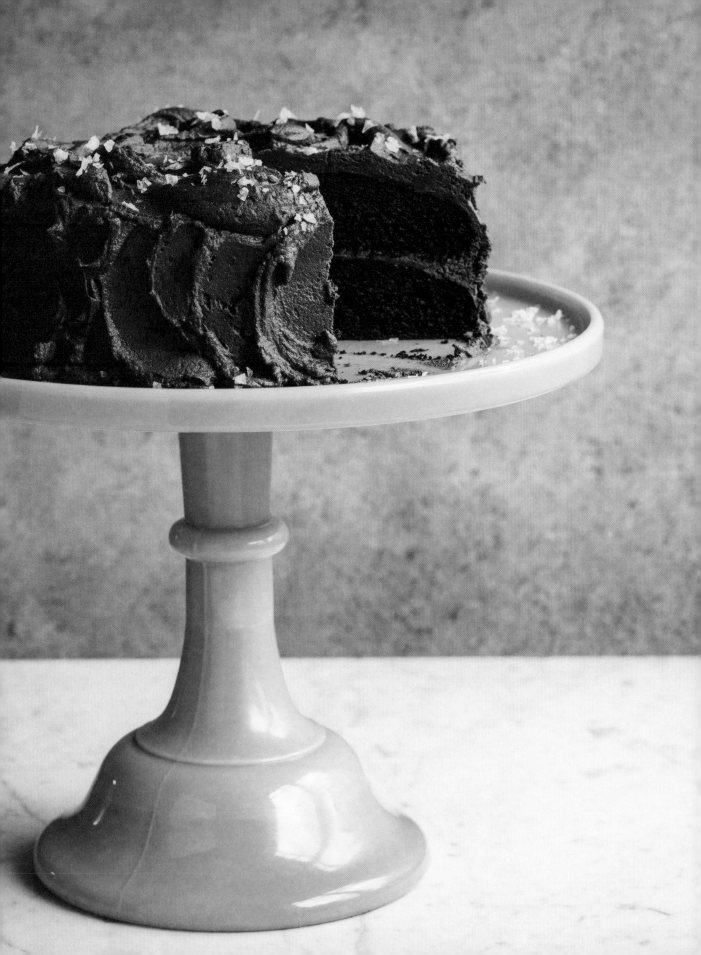

top and sides of the assembled cake with the remaining frosting. Sprinkle with flaky salt, if using. Serve at room temperature.

☆ **MAKE AHEAD**
The cake will keep, covered, in the refrigerator for up to 3 days. Allow the cake to come to room temperature before serving.

NUTRITION INFORMATION (1 PIECE WITH FROSTING):
Calories: 394 | Added sugar: 3¾ teaspoons or 14g | Carbohydrates: 22g | Sodium: 697mg | Saturated fat: 45% of calories or 20g | Fiber: 3g | Protein: 5g

Whipped Chocolate Frosting

◆◆◇◇◇◇◇◇ OURS: 2¼ TEASPOONS
THEIRS: 8 TEASPOONS

Ingredients

10 ounces bittersweet chocolate chips (about 1⅔ cups)
2 cups heavy (whipping) cream
½ teaspoon salt
1 teaspoon pure vanilla extract

MAKES ENOUGH TO FROST AN 8-INCH LAYER CAKE

Whipped dark chocolate frosting adds light layers of creamy chocolate, balancing the intense chocolate cake in our Double Chocolate Layer Cake (page 158). Choose a high-quality dark chocolate for the most flavorful results. Be sure not to overwhip.

1 Place the chocolate chips in the bowl of a stand mixer. Bring the cream and salt to a boil in a medium saucepan over medium heat. Remove from the heat and add the vanilla. Pour the hot cream mixture over the chocolate and allow to sit for 5 minutes, then whisk by hand until completely smooth.

2 Chill, uncovered, in the refrigerator until completely cooled but not hardened, about 1 hour.

3 Fit the stand mixer with a whisk attachment. Attach the bowl with the chocolate mixture. Beat on medium speed until the mixture thickens, about 1 minute. Continue to beat until soft peaks form. Do not overbeat! Use immediately (the frosting will begin to firm up).

NUTRITION INFORMATION (PER SLICE):
Calories: 273 | Added sugar: 2¼ teaspoons or 9g | Carbohydrates: 14g | Sodium: 108mg | Saturated fat: 48% of calories or 14g | Fiber: 5g | Protein: 3g

CHAI-SPICED RICE PUDDING

 OURS = ¾ TEASPOON
THEIRS = 2¼ TEASPOONS

Chai spices add loads of flavor to this remastered version of classic rice pudding. Salted Maple-Date Caramel Sauce subs for sugar and lends the perfect amount of sweetness.

Ingredients

2½ teaspoons ground ginger

1½ teaspoons ground cinnamon

¾ teaspoon ground allspice

¾ teaspoon ground cloves

¼ teaspoon ground cardamom

1 cup medium- or long-grain white rice

3 tablespoons unsalted butter

½ teaspoon salt

3½ cups whole milk

¾ cup Salted Maple-Date Caramel Sauce (page 200)

SERVES 12

1 Combine the ginger, cinnamon, allspice, cloves, and cardamom in a small bowl; set aside.

2 Bring 3 cups water to a boil in a large heavy-bottomed saucepan over medium-high heat. Stir in the rice, 1 tablespoon of the butter, and the salt. Reduce the heat to medium-low and simmer, stirring occasionally, until most of the liquid is absorbed, about 12 minutes.

3 Stir the rice, then stir in the milk, caramel sauce, and spice mixture. Increase the heat to medium-high and bring the mixture to a boil. Reduce the heat to medium-low and simmer, stirring occasionally, until the pudding is thickened and the rice is very tender, 35 to 40 minutes.

4 Remove the rice pudding from the heat. Stir in the remaining 2 tablespoons butter. Serve warm.

VARIATION: Add banana slices and chopped walnuts to turn this pudding into a hearty breakfast.

⭐ **MAKE AHEAD**
The cooled rice pudding will keep in an airtight container in the refrigerator for up to 3 days. Reheat in the microwave with an extra splash of milk, if desired.

NUTRITION INFORMATION (½ CUP):
Calories: 173 | Added sugar: ¾ teaspoon or 3g | Carbohydrates: 27g | Sodium: 140mg | Saturated fat: 17% of calories or 3g | Fiber: 1g | Protein: 4g

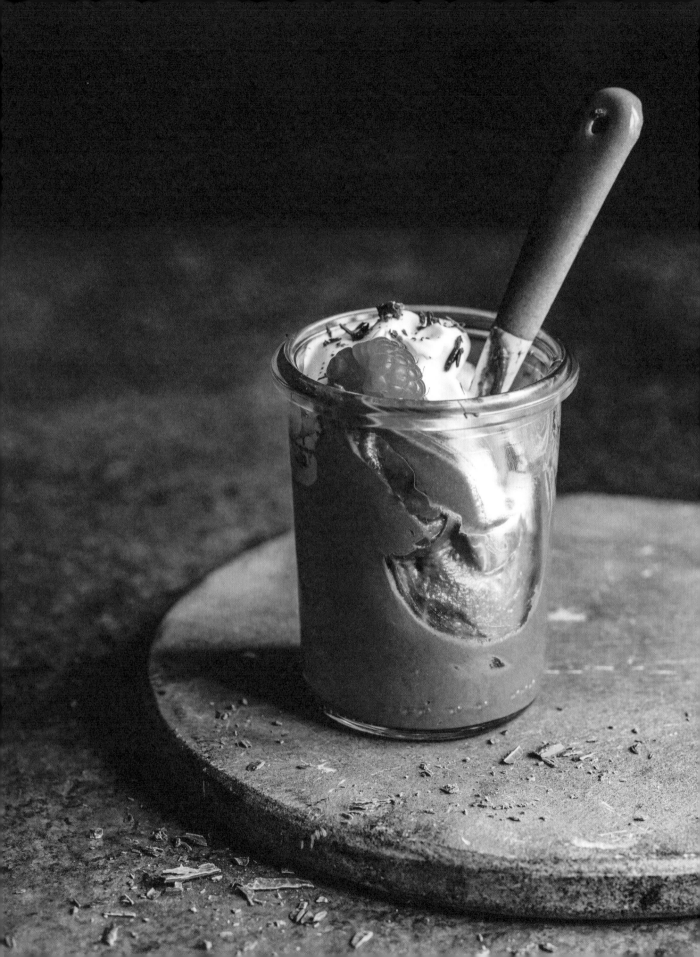

CHOCOLATE PUDDING
WITH MAPLE-VANILLA WHIPPED CREAM

OURS = 1¾ TEASPOONS
THEIRS = 4¼ TEASPOONS

This decadent chocolate pudding is big on flavor and low on added sugar—melted dark chocolate, cocoa powder, and a touch of almond butter add plenty of chocolaty sweetness. Its rich, creamy texture comes from avocado, which also provides a boost of healthy fats. Don't worry—you'll never taste the avocado. Because this pudding is packed with nutritious ingredients and is very rich, the serving size is a little smaller than a packaged pudding cup to keep calories per serving roughly the same. We think you'll find that it's even more satisfying.

1 Place the chocolate chips in a microwave-safe bowl. Microwave in 30-second intervals, stirring in between, until melted, about 1 minute total.

2 Pour the almond milk into a high-powered blender. Add the melted chocolate, cocoa powder, brown sugar, almond butter, vanilla, salt, and avocados and process until smooth and no chunks of avocado remain, about 2 minutes.

3 Cover and chill in the refrigerator for at least 30 minutes.

4 Divide among 10 small cups. Top each with a dollop of the whipped cream and a few fresh raspberries, if using.

☺ **WHAT KIDS CAN DO**
Little chefs can scoop the avocado.

☆ **MAKE AHEAD**
The pudding can be stored, covered, in the refrigerator for up to 2 days.

Ingredients

2 ounces dark chocolate chips (about ⅓ cup)

¾ cup unsweetened almond milk

⅓ cup unsweetened natural cocoa powder

¼ cup packed light brown sugar

2 tablespoons unsweetened almond butter

2 teaspoons pure vanilla extract

½ teaspoon salt

10 to 12 ounces ripe Hass avocado, peeled and pitted (2 small to medium avocados)

Maple-Vanilla Whipped Cream (page 199), for serving (optional)

Fresh raspberries, for serving (optional)

SERVES 10

NUTRITION INFORMATION (ABOUT 2½ OUNCES WITHOUT WHIPPED CREAM):
Calories: 142 | Added sugar: 1¾ teaspoons or 7g | Carbohydrates: 14g | Sodium: 136mg | Saturated fat: 15% of calories or 2g | Fiber: 4g | Protein: 2g

NO-CHURN BANANA ICE CREAM
WITH CHOCOLATE AND SALTED CARAMEL

 OURS = 1½ TEASPOONS
THEIRS: 4 TO 5 TEASPOONS

Ingredients

4 very ripe medium
    bananas, peeled and
    cut into large coins
¼ cup heavy (whipping)
    cream
1 teaspoon pure vanilla
    extract
¼ cup Salted Maple-Date
    Caramel Sauce
    (page 200)
1 ounce dark chocolate,
    shaved with a vegetable
    peeler or grated with
    a grater
Chopped pecans
    (optional)
Dash of flaky sea salt

SERVES 4

☺ WHAT KIDS CAN DO
Kids can slice the
bananas, add the
toppings, and scoop
the ice cream.

☆ MAKE AHEAD
This ice cream can be
stored in the freezer for
2 weeks. Place a layer
of plastic wrap on top,
directly touching the
ice cream, to prevent
freezer burn. Thaw at
room temperature for
20 minutes to soften
before scooping.

This is the easiest ice cream you can make. Simply freeze banana chunks and then whirl them in a food processor. At first they're clumpy, but then suddenly they whip into a creamy ice cream. Mix in some chocolate shavings, caramel, and sweet pecans for a little crunch and freeze briefly to firm it up. You just need to plan ahead by freezing the bananas for at least 6 hours and working quickly once you start the process of making the ice cream. After pureeing, the ice cream will be more "scoopable" if you put it back in the freezer for a couple of hours.

1 Place the banana pieces in a resealable plastic bag in one layer, seal, and freeze until firm, at least 6 hours.

2 Let the bananas thaw for 10 to 15 minutes to soften slightly. Do not leave the bananas out of the freezer much longer or you'll have more of a smoothie than ice cream.

3 Place the banana chunks in a food processor and add the heavy cream and vanilla. Puree until smooth, stopping occasionally to break up large chunks with a spatula, about 5 minutes. At first the bananas will be chunky, but they'll soon smooth out into a custardy frozen treat.

4 Drizzle the caramel sauce over the top and add the chocolate. Pulse once or twice to just barely incorporate the mix-ins. Fold in any unincorporated chocolate shavings and the chopped pecans, if using, with a spatula. To serve, scoop the ice cream into chilled bowls and sprinkle with sea salt. Freeze for 1½ to 2 hours for a firmer texture.

VARIATION: Omit the mix-ins and use just the bananas, cream, vanilla, and salt for an ice cream free of added sugar.

NUTRITION INFORMATION (1 SERVING WITHOUT PECANS):
Calories: 217 | Added sugar: 1½ teaspoons or 6g | Carbohydrates: 41g | Sodium: 53mg | Saturated fat: 15% of calories or 4g | Fiber: 4g | Protein: 2g

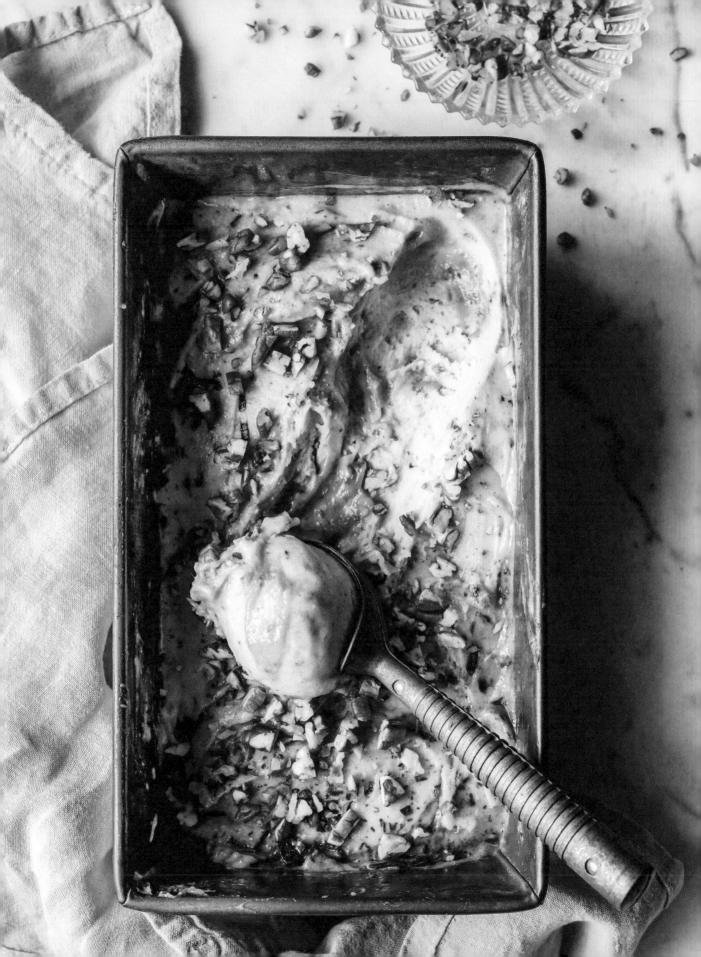

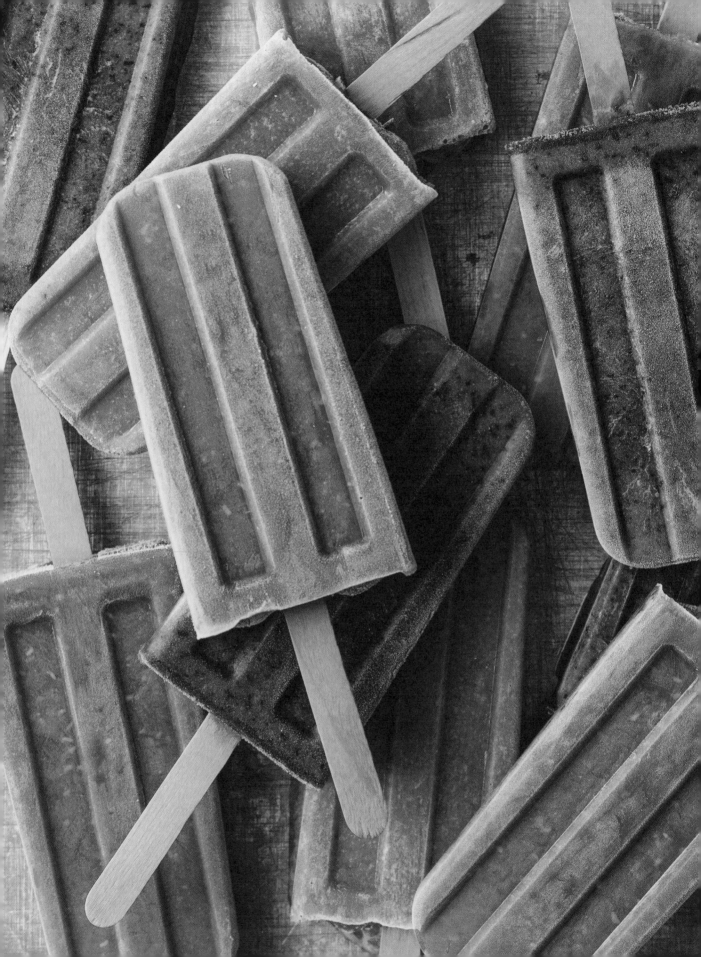

STRAWBERRY CREAM POPS

 OURS = 1 TEASPOON
THEIRS = 2¼ TEASPOONS

Naturally sweet and ripe strawberries make these creamy ice pops a delicious summertime treat. We tried an all-fruit version of these pops but found they were a little too icy and tart. Adding whipping cream and just a touch of sugar helped tremendously with the texture. You will need standard 3-ounce ice pop molds and sticks for these.

Ingredients

1 pound fresh strawberries, hulled and quartered, or 3 cups unsweetened frozen strawberries
2 tablespoons sugar
¼ cup heavy (whipping) cream

MAKES 6 POPS

1 If using frozen fruit, measure what you need and thaw at room temperature until softened, about 30 minutes.

2 Place the fruit and sugar in a blender or food processor and puree until smooth, scraping down the side of the bowl to get any errant chunks. Let sit for 20 minutes to allow the sugar to dissolve. Add the cream and pulse until incorporated.

3 Pour into ice pop molds, up to about ¼ inch from the top, since the mixture expands when frozen. Freeze until thick and slushy, about 30 minutes, then place sticks into the molds. Continue freezing until solid, 4 hours or overnight.

NOTE: If you don't have pop molds, you can use ice cube trays and toothpicks to make about eighteen 1-ounce mini pops. Pour the fruit mixture into ice cube trays, freeze until slushy enough to support the toothpicks, 30 minutes to 1 hour, then add the toothpicks and continue freezing. If using ice cube trays, the added sugar is reduced to about ¼ teaspoon per mini pop.

VARIATION: These pops work equally well with a mixture of berries. Try 1 cup each blueberries, raspberries, and strawberries with the cream and sugar for a triple berry treat.

☺ **WHAT KIDS CAN DO**
Kids can fill the molds.

☆ **MAKE AHEAD**
The pops can be stored, tightly wrapped with plastic wrap, in the freezer for up to 1 month.

NUTRITION INFORMATION (1 STANDARD POP OR 3 MINI POPS):
Calories: 74 | Added sugar: 1 teaspoon or 4g | Carbohydrates: 10g | Sodium: 4mg | Saturated fat: 28% of calories or 2g | Fiber: 2g | Protein: 1g

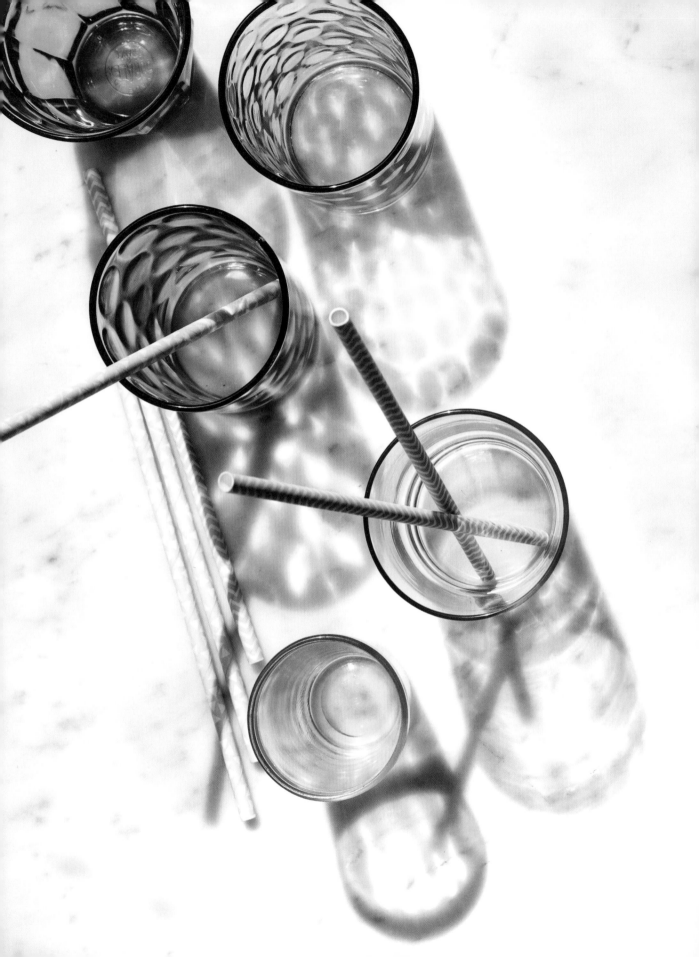

BEVERAGES

Sugar-sweetened beverages are the biggest culprits when it comes to added sugar, contributing nearly 50 percent of total added sugar consumption. Swapping them for something healthier like fruit-infused water or milk is a simple change that will make a big impact. Water is the healthiest drink you can choose, but sometimes you want a treat or a little extra something. These recipes allow you to enjoy your favorites with less sugar and loads of delicious flavor. If you're going to have a sweet drink, make it a healthier one.

CARAMEL COFFEE FRAPPÉ

OURS = 0 TEASPOONS
THEIRS = 5½ TEASPOONS

Ingredients

3 ounces Medjool dates,
    pitted (about 4 dates)

1½ cups hot water

½ cup cold-brew coffee or
    strong brewed coffee,
    at room temperature

½ cup whole milk

½ teaspoon pure vanilla
    extract

8 ice cubes

**MAKES 2 SERVINGS
(8 OUNCES EACH)**

Naturally sweet dates add delicious caramel flavor without the need for added sugar in this sweet and creamy iced coffee. Be sure to fully blend the dates before adding the ice to achieve a super-smooth texture. Caffeine and kids don't mix, so it's best to serve this as an adult beverage—because parents need a treat, too! The chocolaty version (page 171) is for little ones.

1 Place the dates in a medium bowl and cover with the hot water. Soak until very soft, 10 to 15 minutes, then drain.

2 Place the dates in a blender, then add the coffee, milk, and vanilla. Blend on high until the coffee mixture is a consistent color and no flecks of dates remain, 1 to 2 minutes. Add the ice and blend again until smooth, about 1 minute. Serve immediately in tall glasses.

VARIATION: For a more decadent version, use ¼ cup Salted Maple-Date Caramel Sauce (page 200) in place of the dates and vanilla. Blend to break up the ice and then until frothy, about 1 minute. Top with unsweetened whipped cream.

NUTRITION INFORMATION (8 OUNCES):
Calories: 159 | Added sugar: 0 teaspoons or 0g | Carbohydrates: 35g | Sodium: 31mg | Saturated fat: 6% of calories or 1g | Fiber: 3g | Protein: 3g

KIDS' CHOCOLATE FRAPPÉ ⬡

This is similar to the Caramel Coffee Frappé on page 170, but it's a noncaffeinated (and also added sugar–free) version that kids (and adults) will love.

1 Place the dates in a medium bowl and cover with the hot water. Soak until very soft, 10 to 15 minutes, then drain.

2 Combine the cocoa powder and boiling water in a small bowl and stir until the cocoa is dissolved. Let cool for a few minutes.

3 Place the dates, cocoa mixture, milk, and cinnamon in a blender and blend until smooth and no flecks of dates remain, 1 to 2 minutes. Add the ice and blend again until frothy, about 1 minute. Serve immediately in tall glasses, topped with the whipped cream, if you like.

NUTRITION INFORMATION (8 OUNCES):
Calories: 162 | Added sugar: 0 teaspoons or 0g | Carbohydrates: 37g | Sodium: 31mg | Saturated fat: 8% of calories or 1g | Fiber: 4g | Protein: 3g

Ingredients

3 ounces Medjool dates, pitted (about 4 dates)

1½ cups hot water

1 tablespoon unsweetened natural cocoa powder

1 tablespoon boiling water

½ cup whole milk

¼ teaspoon ground cinnamon

8 ice cubes

Maple-Vanilla Whipped Cream (page 199), for serving (optional)

**MAKES 2 SERVINGS
(8 OUNCES EACH)**

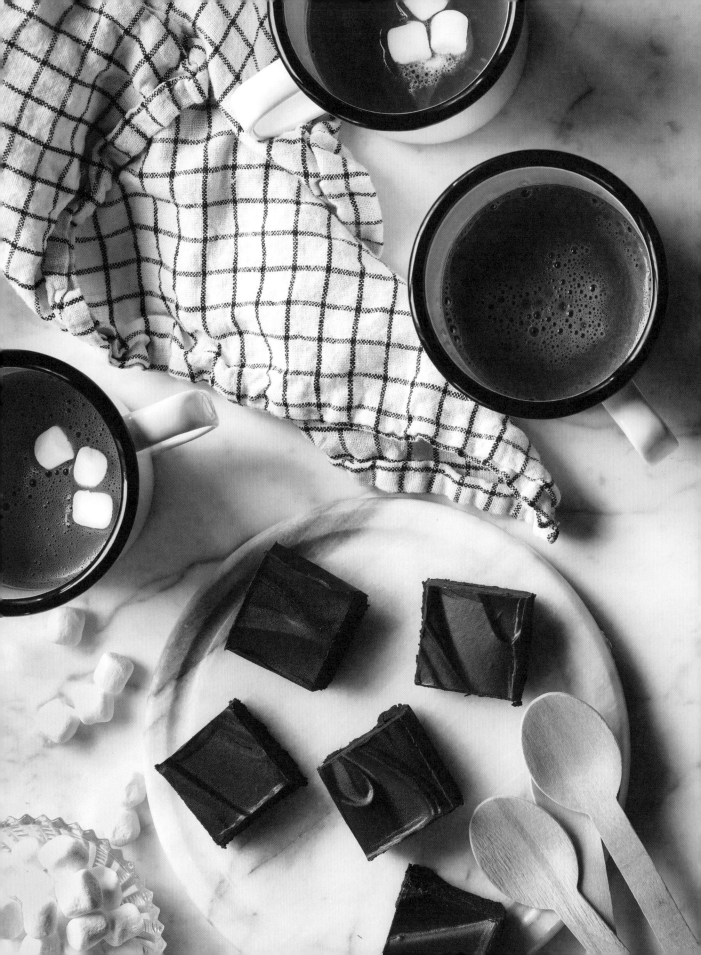

HOT CHOCOLATE BLOCKS

OURS: 2 TEASPOONS
THEIRS: 4 TEASPOONS

This homemade hot chocolate is rich and flavorful thanks to dark chocolate, cream, and a touch of vanilla. Using high-quality dark chocolate results in better flavor so that added sugar can be reduced by 50 percent. Finish off your mug with a few mini marshmallows or a dollop of Maple-Vanilla Whipped Cream for an extra special treat. Wrapped up in a cello bag and tied with a ribbon, these blocks make a lovely teacher gift.

1 Line an 8 × 8-inch baking pan with parchment paper, leaving 2 inches of overhang on each side.

2 Combine the cream, chocolate, vanilla, cinnamon, and salt in a medium heatproof bowl. Set the bowl over a saucepan filled with 1 inch of simmering water over medium heat, making sure the bottom of the bowl doesn't touch the water. Stir until the chocolate is melted and shiny, about 3 minutes.

3 Pour the mixture into the prepared pan. Refrigerate until fully set, 1½ to 2 hours.

4 Remove the chocolate block from the refrigerator. Remove the chocolate from the pan using the parchment paper, transfer to a cutting board, then peel off the parchment paper. Mark the block about every 1½ inches, then cut across four ways and down four ways so you have 25 (1½-inch) squares. Wrap each block in plastic wrap, then place the blocks in a resealable plastic bag and refrigerate or freeze.

5 To serve: For each mug of hot chocolate, pour ¾ cup milk into a small saucepan and bring to a gentle simmer over medium-low heat, 1 to 2 minutes. Be careful not to scorch the milk. Add 1 chocolate block and stir until fully melted. Serve topped with marshmallows, if you like.

☆ **MAKE AHEAD**
The hot chocolate blocks will keep, wrapped, in the refrigerator for up to 1 week or in the freezer for 1 month.

Ingredients

1 cup heavy cream
20 ounces dark chocolate chips (about 3⅓ cups)
1 tablespoon pure vanilla extract
½ teaspoon ground cinnamon
¼ teaspoon salt
Whole milk, for serving
Mini marshmallows or Maple-Vanilla Whipped Cream (page 199), for serving (optional)

MAKES 25 BLOCKS

NUTRITION INFORMATION (1 MUG WITHOUT MARSHMALLOWS OR WHIPPED CREAM):
Calories: 277 | Added sugar: 2 teaspoons or 8g | Carbohydrates: 21g | Sodium: 107mg | Saturated fat: 34% of calories or 11g | Fiber: 2g | Protein: 7g

PUMPKIN SPICE HOT CHOCOLATE

OURS: 1½ TEASPOONS
THEIRS: 4 TEASPOONS

Ingredients

1 teaspoon ground
 cinnamon, plus extra
 for garnish

½ teaspoon sugar

¼ teaspoon ground ginger

¼ teaspoon ground
 nutmeg

¼ teaspoon salt

⅛ teaspoon ground cloves

1 cup heavy (whipping)
 cream

1 tablespoon unsweetened
 natural cocoa powder

2 tablespoons pumpkin
 puree

1 tablespoon pure vanilla
 extract

2 cups whole milk

3 ounces bittersweet
 chocolate chips (½ cup)

Maple-Vanilla Whipped
 Cream (page 199),
 for serving (optional)

SERVES 6

This holiday spiced hot chocolate is a riff on the all-time favorite pumpkin spice latte. Unlike coffee shop versions, this recipe contains real pumpkin puree for a sweet and (little bit) savory sip loaded with flavor. It's a great way to use up those last few scoops of pumpkin when you're making Caramelized Pumpkin Bread (page 51) or Caramelized Pumpkin Pie (page 148).

1 Whisk together the cinnamon, sugar, ginger, nutmeg, salt, and cloves in a small bowl. Set aside.

2 Whisk together the cream and cocoa powder in a medium saucepan over low heat until smooth. Add the spices, pumpkin puree, and vanilla and whisk to fully combine.

3 Add the milk and chocolate chips and bring to a low simmer, stirring constantly, until the chocolate is fully melted. Divide evenly among six mugs and top with the whipped cream, if using, and a dash of cinnamon.

☺ **WHAT KIDS CAN DO**
Kids can stir the cocoa and add the whipped cream.

NUTRITION INFORMATION (1 MUG WITHOUT WHIPPED CREAM):
Calories: 281 | Added sugar: 1½ teaspoons or 6g | Carbohydrates: 15g | Sodium: 145mg | Saturated fat: 45% of calories or 14g | Fiber: 2g | Protein: 5g

HORCHATA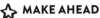

There are many kinds of horchata, a cool cinnamon-rice drink, throughout Latin America. Traditionally, horchata is made with rice soaked in water, or with rice powder or rice flour (which are essentially the same thing, though they can vary in coarseness) mixed with boiling water. Many versions also include dairy milk, sweetened condensed milk, vanilla, and cinnamon. We sweeten ours with dates and swap the condensed milk for unsweetened evaporated milk for thickness.

1 Place the rice, almonds, and dates in a large bowl and cover with 4 cups water. Let soak overnight. Strain, reserving 1½ cups of the soaking liquid.

2 Working in batches if necessary, combine the rice, almonds, and dates in a blender with the reserved soaking liquid and blend until smooth, about 1 minute. Add the whole milk, cinnamon, vanilla, and evaporated milk and blend again until the rice is fully ground, 1 to 2 minutes more.

3 Strain through a fine-mesh strainer and pour into a pitcher. Stir and serve over ice.

☆ **MAKE AHEAD**
The horchata will keep, tightly covered, in the refrigerator, for up to 3 days.

Ingredients

- ¾ cup long-grain white rice
- ¼ cup slivered almonds
- 5 ounces Medjool dates, pitted (about 6 dates)
- 3 cups whole milk
- ½ teaspoon ground cinnamon (preferably canela, aka Mexican cinnamon, if you can find it)
- ¼ teaspoon pure vanilla extract
- 1 can (12 ounces) evaporated milk

MAKES 8 SERVINGS (8 OUNCES EACH)

NUTRITION INFORMATION (8 OUNCES):
Calories: 219 | Added sugar: 0 teaspoons or 0g | Carbohydrates: 30g | Sodium: 90mg | Saturated fat: 16% of calories or 4g | Fiber: 2g | Protein: 8g

STRAWBERRY-CANTALOUPE AGUA FRESCA

OURS: 1 TEASPOON
THEIRS: 3 TEASPOONS

Ingredients

½ cup packed fresh mint leaves, plus a few leaves for garnish (about 8 sprigs fresh mint)

1 tablespoon honey

3 pounds ripe cantaloupe, peeled, seeded, and cut into ½-inch chunks (about 2½ cups)

1 pound strawberries, hulled and sliced (about 2 cups)

1 teaspoon freshly squeezed lemon juice

**MAKES 4 SERVINGS
(12 OUNCES EACH)**

Agua fresca—a refreshing summer drink made with pureed fruit and water—is a staple at most taquerias. Restaurant versions typically add a good amount of sugar to boost flavor, but when ripe, sweet summer fruits are used, there isn't much need for added sugar. This agua fresca uses a simple honey-mint syrup to enhance the natural sweetness of juicy, ripe cantaloupe and height-of-the-season summer strawberries.

1 Combine 1 cup water with the ½ cup mint leaves and the honey in a small saucepan over medium heat. Bring to a gentle boil, stirring occasionally, then reduce the heat to low and simmer until the mint leaves are wilted and the syrup is fragrant, about 5 minutes. Remove from the heat, cover, and let steep for 10 minutes. Strain through a fine-mesh strainer and place in the refrigerator to cool completely, about 30 minutes.

2 Working in batches if necessary, combine the cooled mint syrup, cantaloupe, strawberries, lemon juice, and 2 cups water in a blender and blend on high speed until smooth, about 1 minute. Refrigerate until chilled, at least 30 minutes. Serve over ice, garnished with a few mint leaves.

☆ **MAKE AHEAD**
The agua fresca will keep in an airtight container in the refrigerator for up to 3 days.

NUTRITION INFORMATION (12 OUNCES):
Calories: 83 | Added sugar: 1 teaspoon or 4g | Carbohydrates: 20g | Sodium: 25mg | Saturated fat: 0% of calories or 0g | Fiber: 3g | Protein: 2g

STRAWBERRY-PEACH SMOOTHIE

OURS = 0 TEASPOONS
THEIRS = 8 TO 10 TEASPOONS

This riff on a classic strawberry-banana smoothie gets an extra boost of sweetness from peaches, so you don't have to add the orange or apple juice that you find in commercial versions. Unsweetened cashew milk adds lovely creaminess here, but you can use low-fat dairy milk if you'd prefer.

Working in batches if necessary, combine the milk, strawberries, peaches, and banana in a blender and blend on high until smooth and creamy, about 1 minute. Serve immediately.

☺ **WHAT KIDS CAN DO**
Kids can measure the ingredients and load them into the blender.

NUTRITION INFORMATION (16 OUNCES):
Calories: 130 | Added sugar: 0 teaspoons or 0g | Carbohydrates: 28g | Sodium: 162mg | Saturated fat: 0% of calories or 0g | Fiber: 4g | Protein: 2g

Ingredients

2 cups unsweetened cashew milk or low-fat milk
5 ounces frozen strawberries (about 1 cup)
5 ounces frozen peaches (about 1 cup)
1 large banana, peeled, frozen, and cut into 4 large chunks

MAKES 2 SERVINGS (16 OUNCES EACH)

MANGO-PINEAPPLE SMOOTHIE ⊗

OURS: 0 TEASPOONS
THEIRS: 8 TO 10 TEASPOONS

Ingredients

1½ cups coconut milk or
low-fat milk

5 ounces frozen pineapple
(about 1 cup)

5 ounces frozen mango
(about 1 cup)

1 large banana, peeled,
frozen, and cut into
4 large chunks

⅔ cup low-fat plain Greek
yogurt or coconut
yogurt

**MAKES 2 SERVINGS
(16 OUNCES EACH)**

This tropical fruit smoothie gets its sweetness from pineapples and mango instead of the sweetened frozen yogurt, sherbet, or juice that is typically found in restaurant versions of this drink. Blending this smoothie with coconut milk maximizes its piña colada flavor, but the recipe works equally well with low-fat dairy milk.

Working in batches if necessary, combine the milk, pineapple, mango, banana, and yogurt in a blender and blend on high until smooth and creamy, about 1 minute. Serve immediately.

☺ **WHAT KIDS CAN DO**
Kids can measure the ingredients and load them into the blender.

NUTRITION INFORMATION (16 OUNCES):
Calories: 266 | Added sugar: 0 teaspoons or 0g | Carbohydrates: 47g | Sodium: 109mg | Saturated fat: 7% of calories or 2g | Fiber: 4g | Protein: 15g

Refreshing low-sugar smoothies (from left to right):
Strawberry-Peach Smoothie (page 177),
Blueberry-Almond Smoothie (page 181),
Mango-Pineapple Smoothie (page 178)

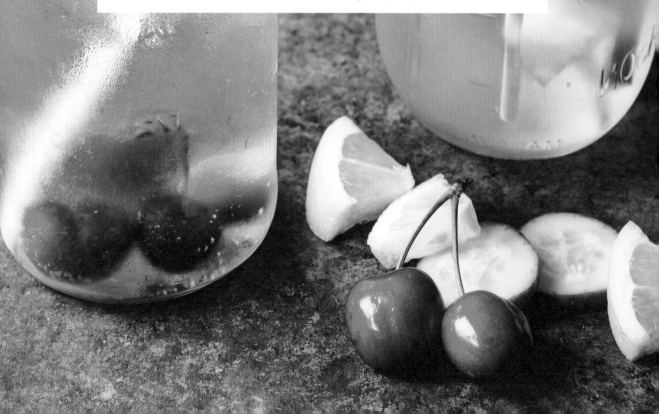

DRINK WATER!

To make water fun and flavorful, add fresh fruits, vegetables, and herbs to a pitcher of chilled water. You can also freeze chopped fruits and veggies with water in an ice-cube tray to add fun pops of color to your drinks.

Here are some of our favorite combinations:
• Lemon, lime, orange
• Strawberry, lemon, basil
• Cucumber, lime
• Watermelon, mint
• Mango, raspberry

BLUEBERRY-ALMOND SMOOTHIE ⊗

▢▢▢▢▢▢▢▢▢▢ OURS: 0 TEASPOONS
THEIRS: 8 TO 10 TEASPOONS

This sweet, creamy, and satisfying smoothie is made without dairy or juice. Blueberries and bananas give it loads of natural sweetness, and its creaminess comes from a touch of almond butter. It makes a great breakfast for kids (and adults!) when you are in a rush to head out the door in the morning.

Working in batches if necessary, combine the milk, blueberries, banana, and almond butter in a blender and blend on high until smooth and creamy, about 1 minute. Serve immediately.

☺ **WHAT KIDS CAN DO**
Kids can measure the ingredients and load them into the blender.

NUTRITION INFORMATION (16 OUNCES):
Calories: 262 | Added sugar: 0 teaspoons or 0g | Carbohydrates: 35g | Sodium: 224mg | Saturated fat: 4% of calories or 1g | Fiber: 7g | Protein: 6g

Ingredients

2 cups unsweetened almond milk

10 ounces frozen blueberries (about 2 cups)

1 large banana, peeled, frozen, and cut into 4 equal chunks

2 tablespoons unsweetened almond butter

MAKES 2 SERVINGS (16 OUNCES EACH)

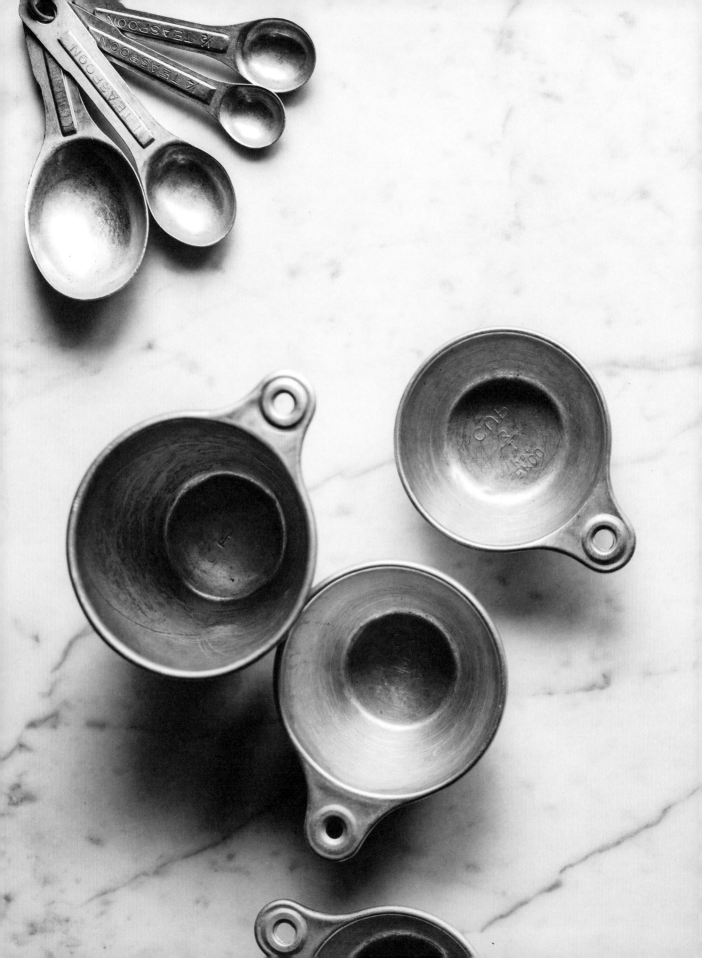

BASICS AND CONDIMENTS

Popular bottled sauces such as teriyaki and BBQ can contain a sneaky amount of hidden sugars. This is also true of kid-favorite condiments like ketchup, sweet spreads, and dessert sauces. Some salad dressings hide a surprising amount of added sugar, too. We've remastered your favorites with half the sugar—and sometimes no sugar at all. Many of the recipes in the Dinners chapter (page 91) make clever use of our Big Batch Sauces (pages 185–189), which can be made ahead of time and stored in the refrigerator. (They are marked with a ▢ icon so they're easy to spot.) It's a great idea to do the same with other basics and condiments so you'll always have them on hand.

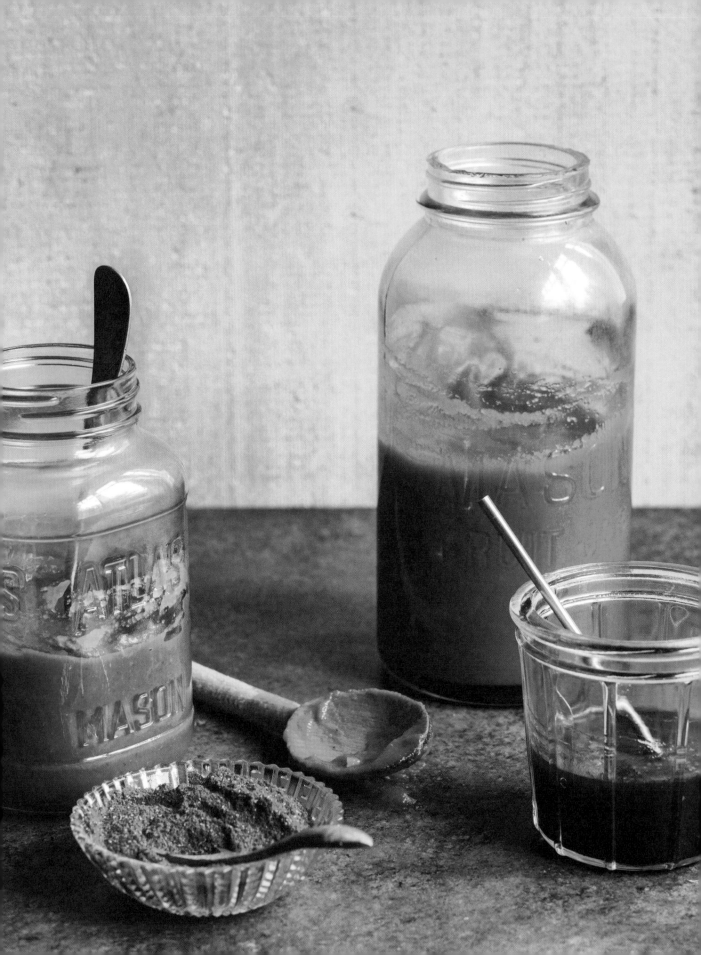

BBQ SAUCE AND SPICE MIX

Sweet onions and nectarines—as well as the more unusual but delicious addition of unsweetened cocoa powder—give this sauce a natural sweetness. Added sugar in packaged BBQ sauces varies widely, from a whopping 4 teaspoons per serving to 2 to 3 teaspoons in most brands. Our sauce contains just ¾ teaspoon per serving. This recipe makes extra sauce as well as an all-purpose spice mix for seasoning pulled pork (see page 105), chicken (see page 96), ribs, or other meats.

1 Make the spice mix: Combine the cocoa powder, ginger, salt, paprika, chipotle chile powder, garlic, thyme, and pepper in a small bowl.

2 Make the sauce: Heat the oil in a large saucepan over medium-low heat. Add the onion and sauté until very tender, 12 to 15 minutes, stirring often.

3 Add 3 tablespoons of the spice mix (reserve the rest in an airtight container) and stir into the onion mix. Add the sugar, vinegar, nectarines, and tomato paste plus 1½ cups water. Stir well, scraping the bottom of the pan, and bring to a simmer. Reduce the heat to low and cook until thickened, 20 to 30 minutes. Puree until smooth with an immersion blender, or let cool, then puree in a blender.

NOTE: Smoked paprika and chipotle chile powder can make the sauce a bit spicy. For a milder sauce, substitute liquid smoke, starting with 1 teaspoon, then adding more to taste.

⚡ QUICK TIP
Combine 1 cup bottled BBQ sauce (preferably one with 12 grams of sugar or less per serving) with 1¼ cups strained or pureed tomatoes in a small saucepan with 1 to 2 teaspoons hot sauce and a dash of black pepper. Bring to a simmer, then reduce the heat to low and cook, stirring occasionally, until the sauce thickens, 5 to 10 minutes. This will increase the added sugar to 1½ to 2 teaspoons per serving.

☆ MAKE AHEAD
The spice mix will keep in an airtight container away from light and heat for several months. The sauce will keep in a jar or airtight container in the refrigerator for up to 1 month.

Ingredients

FOR THE SPICE MIX

2 tablespoons unsweetened natural cocoa powder

2 teaspoons ground ginger

2 teaspoons salt

1½ to 3 teaspoons smoked paprika (see Note)

1 to 2 teaspoons chipotle chile powder (see Note) or chili powder

1 teaspoon granulated garlic

1 teaspoon dried thyme

½ teaspoon freshly ground black pepper

FOR THE BBQ SAUCE

2 tablespoons vegetable oil

2 cups chopped sweet onion (1 large onion)

⅓ cup packed light brown sugar

3 tablespoons apple cider vinegar

2 nectarines, pitted and chopped, or 10 ounces frozen peaches, thawed, drained, and chopped

1 can (6 ounces) tomato paste

MAKES 3½ CUPS BBQ SAUCE AND ABOUT 6 TABLESPOONS SPICE MIX

NUTRITION INFORMATION (2 TABLESPOONS SAUCE):
Calories: 34 | Added sugar: ¾ teaspoon or 3g | Carbohydrates: 6g | Sodium: 89mg | Saturated fat: 3% of calories or 1g | Fiber: 1g | Protein: 1g

PINEAPPLE TERIYAKI GLAZE

OURS = ¼ TEASPOON
THEIRS = 1¾ TEASPOONS

Ingredients

1¼ cups low-sodium
   soy sauce
1 cup sake
1 cup finely chopped
   pineapple
¼ cup plus 1 tablespoon
   packed dark brown
   sugar
1 tablespoon finely
   chopped garlic
1 teaspoon peeled and
   finely grated fresh
   ginger

MAKES 3 CUPS

Teriyaki sauce was originally a simple glaze for grilled meats made with soy sauce, rice wine, and a little sugar. But it's gotten sweeter over the years, especially in commercial bottled sauces, with new add-ins like ginger, garlic, and sesame seeds. This version has all the flavor of those with less added sugar, thanks to the pineapple.

1 Place the soy sauce, sake, pineapple, brown sugar, garlic, ginger, and 1 cup water in a small saucepan. Bring to a simmer, stirring occasionally, and then reduce the heat and cook until reduced slightly and the flavors have come together, about 20 minutes. Let cool briefly.

2 Puree in a blender or food processor.

☆ **MAKE AHEAD**
The glaze will keep in a jar or airtight container in the refrigerator for up to 1 month.

NUTRITION INFORMATION (1 TABLESPOON):
Calories: 19 | Added sugar: ¼ teaspoon or 1g | Carbohydrates: 3g | Sodium: 222mg | Saturated fat: 0% of calories or 0g | Fiber: 0g | Protein: 0g

CHINESE HOISIN SAUCE 🫙

OURS = ¼ TEASPOON
THEIRS = 2¼ TEASPOONS

The ultra-sweet, gloopy hoisin sauce used in many Chinese dishes and marinades can taste like candy. This version is less thick and cloying but still has a sweet-salty balance and the captivating flavor of Chinese five-spice powder, which is easy to find online or in grocery stores with decent spice sections. If you have trouble finding miso paste, unsweetened natural peanut butter is a great substitute here.

1 Combine the soy sauce, vinegar, sesame oil, garlic, sugar, red pepper flakes, black pepper, and five-spice powder in a small saucepan. Bring to a simmer over medium-low heat and stir to melt the sugar, 1 minute. Reduce the heat to low and stir in the miso paste. Bring to a gentle simmer.

2 Place the cornstarch in a small bowl, stir in 2 tablespoons water, then add this slurry to the sauce, and simmer until slightly thickened, about 30 seconds. Let cool completely.

⭐ **MAKE AHEAD**
The sauce will keep in a jar or airtight container in the refrigerator for up to 1 month.

NUTRITION INFORMATION (2 TABLESPOONS):
Calories: 54 | Added sugar: ¼ teaspoon or 1g | Carbohydrates: 6g | Sodium: 923mg | Saturated fat: 7% of calories or 1g | Fiber: 0g | Protein: 2g

Ingredients

1 cup low-sodium soy sauce or tamari

3 tablespoons unseasoned rice vinegar

2 tablespoons toasted (dark) sesame oil

2 tablespoons finely minced garlic

4 teaspoons sugar

1 teaspoon crushed red pepper flakes or chili oil

½ teaspoon freshly ground black pepper

½ teaspoon Chinese five-spice powder

¼ cup white miso paste

1 tablespoon cornstarch

MAKES ABOUT 1½ CUPS

QUICK-COOK TOMATO-BASIL SAUCE ⬢ ▯

OURS = 0 TEASPOONS
THEIRS = ½ TEASPOON

Ingredients

2 tablespoons extra-virgin olive oil

1 tablespoon finely chopped garlic

¼ teaspoon crushed red pepper flakes

¼ teaspoon dried oregano

2 cans (28 ounces each) low-sodium strained tomatoes or tomato puree

1 teaspoon salt, plus extra as needed

4 large fresh basil leaves, torn

MAKES 5 CUPS

Tomato sauce is one of the sneaky places where added sugar lurks—it's used to sweeten less-than-ripe tomatoes and as a preservative for longer shelf life. Making sauce at home is the easiest way to control the sugar in this family staple. Homemade sauce can be a time-consuming endeavor, but it doesn't have to be. This quick-cook sauce takes only about 20 minutes to make. The recipe makes enough for Rainbow Chard Lasagna (page 121) or Spinach-Ricotta Calzones (page 127). Using strained tomatoes makes the sauce easy to prepare and the perfect consistency for lasagna and other pasta dishes.

1 Heat a large skillet over medium-low heat and add the olive oil. When it is warm, add the garlic, red pepper flakes, and oregano and swirl in the oil until just fragrant, about 30 seconds.

2 Add the tomatoes and salt. Bring to a low boil, then reduce the heat to low and simmer, stirring occasionally, until the tomatoes have lost their raw flavor and the sauce is sweeter, about 20 minutes.

3 Stir in the basil and adjust the seasoning to taste.

☆ **MAKE AHEAD**
The sauce will keep in a jar or airtight container in the refrigerator for 1 week or in the freezer for 3 months. If frozen, thaw the sauce overnight in the refrigerator.

NUTRITION INFORMATION (½ CUP):
Calories: 66 | Added sugar: 0 teaspoons or 0g | Carbohydrates: 9g | Sodium: 246mg | Saturated fat: 5% of calories or 1g | Fiber: 3g | Protein: 0g

SLOW-COOKER TOMATO-BASIL SAUCE

OURS = 0 TEASPOONS*
THEIRS = ½ TEASPOON

Strained tomatoes help to produce a smooth, consistent texture with no seeds in this slow-cooker sauce. A touch of sugar is stirred in to reduce acidity, but it adds a negligible amount per serving.

1 Place the tomatoes in a slow cooker.

2 Heat a large skillet over medium-low heat and add the olive oil. When warm, add the marjoram and swirl in the oil for a few seconds. Add the onion and cook over low heat until tender but not browned, stirring often, about 10 minutes. Add the garlic and cook until its flavor begins to infuse the sauce, about 2 more minutes.

3 Add the wine and stir, scraping the bottom of the pan to incorporate any browned bits. Simmer to reduce slightly, about 2 minutes.

4 Scrape the contents of the pan into the slow cooker with a silicone spatula, then add the parsley, salt, sugar, and basil and stir together.

5 Cover and cook on high for 6 hours or on low for 12 hours.

6 Uncover and remove and discard the garlic cloves. Add the butter and stir until the butter is melted, then adjust the seasoning to taste.

QUICK TIP
To make a chunky sauce, use 2 cans (28 ounces each) whole peeled tomatoes instead of strained tomatoes. Place the whole peeled tomatoes with their juices into the slow cooker and squeeze with clean hands to roughly shred the tomatoes. Then proceed with Step 2.

MAKE AHEAD
The sauce will keep in a jar or airtight container in the refrigerator for 1 week or in the freezer for 3 months. If frozen, thaw the sauce overnight in the refrigerator.

Ingredients

- 2 cans (28 ounces each) low-sodium strained tomatoes or tomato puree
- 2 tablespoons extra-virgin olive oil
- ½ teaspoon dried marjoram
- 1 large sweet onion, peeled and finely diced (about 1 cup)
- 3 cloves garlic, peeled and lightly crushed
- ¼ cup dry red wine
- ½ cup finely chopped fresh flat-leaf (Italian) parsley (about ½ bunch)
- 1 teaspoon salt
- 1 teaspoon sugar
- 4 sprigs fresh basil, stems removed
- 1 tablespoon unsalted butter

MAKES ABOUT 5 CUPS

NUTRITION INFORMATION (½ CUP):
Calories: 70 | Added sugar: 0 teaspoons or 0g | Carbohydrates: 7g | Sodium: 242mg | Saturated fat: 14% of calories or 1g | Fiber: 2g | Protein: <1g

*Negligible

KETCHUP

OURS = ¼ TEASPOON
THEIRS = ¾ TEASPOON

Ingredients

1½ ounces pitted
   Deglet Noor dates
   (5 to 6 dates)
1 cup hot water
1 tablespoon extra-virgin
   olive oil
1 cup finely chopped sweet
   onion
2 tablespoons white
   vinegar
1 tablespoon packed dark
   brown sugar
1 teaspoon Worcestershire
   sauce
¾ teaspoon salt
¼ teaspoon freshly ground
   black pepper
3 ounces tomato paste
   (½ of a 6-ounce can)

MAKES 1 CUP

The combination of gently sautéed sweet onions, dates, and a touch of brown sugar adds just enough sweetness to this typically sugar-laden condiment. Tomato paste provides rich, concentrated tomato flavor, while white vinegar gives the sauce clean, lip-smacking tartness. This homemade ketchup will be lighter in color than the store-bought versions. The shortcut version of this recipe is great in a pinch. Although not as low in sugar as the from-scratch version, it's equally delicious.

1 Place the dates in a medium bowl and cover with the hot water. Let the dates soak for 10 minutes.

2 Meanwhile, heat the oil in a small saucepan over medium-low heat. Add the onion and sauté until very tender, stirring often, 12 to 15 minutes.

3 Add the dates and their soaking liquid, vinegar, brown sugar, Worcestershire sauce, salt, pepper, and tomato paste to the saucepan. Bring to a simmer over medium-high heat, stirring occasionally.

4 Reduce the heat to medium-low and cook until thickened, about 20 minutes. Stir in ¼ cup water. Let the mixture cool for 10 minutes before transferring to a blender. Blend until smooth, 1 minute.

5 Transfer the ketchup to an airtight container and refrigerate until completely chilled before serving.

⚡ QUICK TIP
Combine ½ cup bottled ketchup (preferably one with 4 grams sugar or less per serving), ½ cup pureed tomatoes, 1 teaspoon white vinegar, and ½ teaspoon onion powder in a small saucepan. Bring to a simmer over medium-high heat, then lower the heat to low and cook until the ketchup thickens and the flavors combine, stirring occasionally, about 5 minutes. This will increase the added sugar to about ⅓ teaspoon per serving.

☆ MAKE AHEAD
The ketchup will keep in a jar or airtight container in the refrigerator for up to 2 weeks.

NUTRITION INFORMATION (1 TABLESPOON):
Calories: 27 | Added sugar: ¼ teaspoon or 1g | Carbohydrates: 5g | Sodium: 116mg | Saturated fat: 3% of calories or <1g | Fiber: 1g | Protein: <1g

CRANBERRY SAUCE

 OURS: ¼ TEASPOON
THEIRS: 2½ TEASPOONS

Pureed frozen peaches and dried apricots—along with a small amount of granulated sugar—mellow out the tartness of the cranberries in this rustic sauce.

1 Place the apricots in a small bowl and cover with the hot water. Let soak for 5 minutes.

2 Finely grate the zest of half the orange (you should have about 1½ teaspoons) and transfer to a small saucepan. Reserve the orange for another use.

3 Place the softened apricots and their soaking liquid in a blender. Add the peach slices and blend until mostly smooth, with some visible apricot flecks, about 1 minute, stopping the blender as needed to scrape down the sides. Transfer the mixture to the saucepan.

4 Add the cranberries and sugar to the saucepan and bring to a boil over medium-high heat. Reduce the heat to medium-low and simmer, stirring occasionally, until the cranberries start to burst, about 3 minutes.

5 Continue cooking until the cranberries break down and the mixture thickens, about 5 minutes, using a spatula to stir occasionally.

6 Transfer the cranberry sauce to a heatproof bowl and let cool completely. Cover and refrigerate until ready to use.

☆ **MAKE AHEAD**
The cranberry sauce will keep in a jar or airtight container in the refrigerator for up to 1 week.

Ingredients

2 ounces dried apricots
  (about ¼ cup or
  8 to 10 pieces)
¼ cup hot water
1 navel orange
½ cup frozen peach slices
  (about 5 slices)
1½ cups fresh or frozen
  cranberries
1 tablespoon sugar

**MAKES 1 CUP PLUS
2 TABLESPOONS**

NUTRITION INFORMATION (2 TABLESPOONS):
Calories: 41 | Added sugar: ¼ teaspoon or 1g | Carbohydrates: 11g | Sodium: 1mg | Saturated fat: 0% of calories or 0g | Fiber: 2g | Protein: <1g

CREAMY RANCH DRESSING

OURS = 0 TEASPOONS*
THEIRS = ¼ TEASPOON

Ingredients

2 tablespoons white wine vinegar

2 teaspoons finely chopped fresh chives (optional)

1 teaspoon dried dill or 1 tablespoon finely chopped fresh dill

½ teaspoon garlic powder

½ teaspoon onion powder

½ teaspoon sugar

½ teaspoon salt

¼ teaspoon freshly ground black pepper, plus extra as needed

½ cup plus 2 tablespoons whole milk plain Greek yogurt

MAKES ABOUT 1 CUP

Dried spices add loads of flavor to this quick and easy ranch dressing. It can be used as a dip for your favorite sliced veggies or as a dressing for BBQ Chicken Chopped Salad (page 87).

Whisk together the vinegar, chives, if using, dill, garlic powder, onion powder, sugar, salt, and pepper in a medium bowl. Whisk in the yogurt and season to taste with more pepper if needed.

⭐ **MAKE AHEAD**
The dressing will keep in a jar or airtight container in the refrigerator for 1 week.

NUTRITION INFORMATION (2 TABLESPOONS):
Calories: 21 | Added sugar: 0 teaspoons or 0g | Carbohydrates: 1g | Sodium: 152mg | Saturated fat: 0% of calories or <0.5g | Fiber: 0g | Protein: 2g

*Negligible

MANDARIN VINAIGRETTE

OURS = 0 TEASPOONS
THEIRS = 2 TEASPOONS

Tangy mandarin oranges, toasted sesame oil, and a touch of ginger create a quick and easy salad dressing for our Chinese Chicken Salad (page 85). The bright and fresh flavor is one that kids typically like, making it a good option for getting reluctant eaters to enjoy salad.

Whisk together the mandarin juice, vinegar, soy sauce, garlic, ginger, and salt in a medium bowl. Slowly drizzle in the oils while whisking until incorporated. Season to taste with more salt, vinegar, and/or sesame oil.

NOTE: If you can't find a mandarin orange, substitute a tangerine or a clementine instead.

⭐ **MAKE AHEAD**
The vinaigrette will keep in a jar or airtight container in the refrigerator for 1 week.

NUTRITION INFORMATION (2 TABLESPOONS):
Calories: 92 | Added sugar: 0 teaspoons or 0g | Carbohydrates: 2g | Sodium: 94mg | Saturated fat: 10% of calories or 1g | Fiber: <1g | Protein: <1g

Ingredients

½ cup freshly squeezed mandarin orange juice (see Note)

¼ cup apple cider vinegar or white wine vinegar, plus extra as needed

2 teaspoons low-sodium soy sauce

1½ teaspoons finely minced garlic

1 teaspoon peeled and finely grated fresh ginger

¼ teaspoon salt, plus extra as needed

¼ cup vegetable oil

3 tablespoons toasted (dark) sesame oil, plus extra as needed

MAKES 1¼ CUPS

CREAMY POPPY SEED DRESSING

OURS = ¼ TEASPOON
THEIRS = 1¾ TEASPOONS

Ingredients

1 medium very ripe
   Bartlett pear (about
   7 ounces), cored and
   diced (skin left on)
¼ cup extra-virgin olive oil
3 tablespoons white wine
   vinegar
1 tablespoon finely
   chopped shallot
2 teaspoons Dijon
   mustard
2 teaspoons honey
¼ teaspoon salt
¼ teaspoon freshly ground
   black pepper
1½ teaspoons poppy seeds

MAKES 1 CUP

A typical store-bought creamy poppy seed dressing has almost
2 teaspoons of added sugar per serving. The addition of a ripe pear
gives this typically sugar-laden dressing the bulk of its sweetness,
as well as a rich and creamy consistency without the need for milk.

1 Place the pear, oil, vinegar,
   shallot, mustard, honey, salt,
and pepper in a blender. Blend
until smooth and creamy, about
1 minute.

2 Add the poppy seeds and pulse
   to combine. Transfer the
dressing to an airtight container
and refrigerate until ready to use.

⭐ **MAKE AHEAD**
The dressing will keep in a jar or
airtight container in the refrigerator
for up to 3 days.

NUTRITION INFORMATION (2 TABLESPOONS):
Calories: 85 | Added sugar: ¼ teaspoon or 1g | Carbohydrates: 6g | Sodium: 88mg |
Saturated fat: 11% of calories or 1g | Fiber: 1g | Protein: 0g

ROASTED STRAWBERRY BALSAMIC VINAIGRETTE ⊗

Slow-roasting the strawberries helps draw out excess moisture while concentrating their flavor and sweetness. A combination of syrupy balsamic vinegar and tart red wine vinegar brings balance to this zingy fruit-based vinaigrette.

Ingredients

6 ounces strawberries, hulled and quartered, (about 1 cup)

3 tablespoons extra-virgin olive oil

1 tablespoon balsamic vinegar

1 tablespoon red wine vinegar

¼ teaspoon salt

¼ teaspoon freshly ground black pepper

MAKES ½ CUP

1 Preheat the oven to 350°F.

2 Toss the strawberries and 1 tablespoon of the oil in a pie plate. Roast until the strawberries are softened and appear glazed, about 20 minutes, stirring once halfway through baking. Set the strawberries aside to cool for 10 minutes.

3 Place the strawberries, the remaining 2 tablespoons oil, the balsamic vinegar, red wine vinegar, salt, and pepper in a blender. Blend until smooth, about 1 minute.

4 Transfer the vinaigrette to an airtight container and refrigerate until ready to use.

☆ **MAKE AHEAD**
The vinaigrette will keep in a jar or airtight container in the refrigerator for up to 3 days.

NUTRITION INFORMATION (2 TABLESPOONS):
Calories: 108 | Added sugar: 0 teaspoons or 0g | Carbohydrates: 4g | Sodium: 147mg | Saturated fat: 12% of calories or 1g | Fiber: 1g | Protein: <1g

NEWTELLA

OURS = 1 TEASPOON
THEIRS = 4¾ TEASPOONS

Ingredients

1 cup raw hazelnuts,
skin on
1 ounce unsweetened
chocolate, finely
chopped (about 3
tablespoons)
3 tablespoons
confectioners' sugar
1 tablespoon unsweetened
natural cocoa powder
1 tablespoon vegetable oil
½ teaspoon pure vanilla
extract
¼ teaspoon salt

MAKES ¾ CUP

Inspired by the ubiquitous Italian chocolate-hazelnut spread, this remastered version satisfies all your cravings for a chocolaty snack with a fraction of the added sugar. Toasted hazelnuts provide rich, deep flavor that's rounded out with unsweetened chocolate and a touch of vanilla.

1 Preheat the oven to 350°F.

2 Place the hazelnuts on a rimmed baking sheet and toast until the skins are dark brown and have started to blister, 10 to 12 minutes, rotating the baking sheet 180 degrees halfway through baking.

3 Wrap the hazelnuts in a clean kitchen towel and rub to remove the loose skins; discard the skins. Transfer the nuts to a food processor and process until they form a thick paste, about 4 minutes, stopping occasionally to scrape the bottom and side of the bowl.

4 Meanwhile, place the chocolate in a microwave-safe bowl and microwave in 20-second intervals, stirring after each interval, until melted, about 1 minute total.

5 Add the confectioners' sugar, cocoa powder, oil, vanilla, and salt to the hazelnut paste and process until smooth, about 1 minute. Scrape down the bowl.

6 Add the melted chocolate and process until combined, about 1 minute.

7 Transfer the mixture to a jar or an airtight container and let it cool to room temperature before using.

☺ WHAT KIDS CAN DO
Little chefs can rub the toasted hazelnuts in a kitchen towel to remove their skins (be careful, as they might be hot) and load the ingredients into the food processor.

☆ MAKE AHEAD
The spread will keep in a jar or airtight container in the refrigerator for up to 2 weeks. Let it come to room temperature before using.

NUTRITION INFORMATION (2 TABLESPOONS):
Calories: 212 | Added sugar: 1 teaspoon or 4g | Carbohydrates: 10g | Sodium: 98mg | Saturated fat: 12% of calories or 3g | Fiber: 3g | Protein: 4g

NUT-FREE NEWTELLA

OURS = ½ TEASPOON
THEIRS = 4¾ TEASPOONS

This nut-free version of our chocolate-hazelnut spread (see page 196) is a great option for kids with allergies or those who tote a packed lunch to a school that is nut-free. This spread is loaded with delicious flavor and healthy fats from pumpkin and sunflower seeds, and it uses a fraction of the sugar of the store-bought equivalent. It makes a great teacher gift.

1 Place the sunflower seeds and pumpkin seeds in a food processor. Process until a cohesive paste forms, about 3 minutes. Scrape the bottom and side of the bowl. Continue processing until smooth, about 3 minutes more, stopping after every minute to scrape down the bowl.

2 Place the chocolate in a microwave-safe bowl and microwave in 20-second intervals, stirring after each interval, until melted, about 1 minute total.

3 Add the confectioners' sugar, cocoa powder, oil, and salt to the seed paste and process until the mixture is smooth, about 1 minute. Stop to scrape down the bowl.

4 Add the melted chocolate and process until combined, about 1 minute.

5 Transfer the mixture to a jar or airtight container and let it cool to room temperature before using.

☺ **WHAT KIDS CAN DO**
Little ones can measure the ingredients.

☆ **MAKE AHEAD**
The spread will keep in a jar or airtight container in the refrigerator for up to 2 weeks. Let it come to room temperature before using.

Ingredients

½ cup roasted unsalted sunflower seeds
½ cup roasted unsalted pumpkin seeds
1 ounce unsweetened chocolate, finely chopped (about 3 tablespoons)
2 tablespoons confectioners' sugar
1 tablespoon unsweetened natural cocoa powder
1 tablespoon vegetable oil
¼ teaspoon salt

MAKES ¾ CUP

NUTRITION INFORMATION (2 TABLESPOONS):
Calories: 183 | Added sugar: ½ teaspoon or 2g | Carbohydrates: 9g | Sodium: 100mg | Saturated fat: 16% of calories or 3g | Fiber: 3g | Protein: 6g

THREE-INGREDIENT STRAWBERRY JAM

OURS: ¼ TEASPOON
THEIRS: 2½ TEASPOONS

Ingredients

9 ounces strawberries,
   hulled and sliced
   (about 1½ cups)
¼ cup unsweetened
   applesauce
1 tablespoon sugar

MAKES ¾ CUP

This small-batch strawberry jam comes together quickly and contains very little added sugar. A bit of unsweetened applesauce adds natural sweetness and helps bind the cooked strawberries together into a slightly chunky yet spreadable jam.

1 Stir together the strawberries, applesauce, and sugar in a small saucepan. Bring to a simmer over medium-high heat, 1 minute.

2 Reduce the heat to medium and continue to cook, stirring occasionally, until most of the strawberries break down and the mixture thickens, 13 to 15 minutes.

3 Transfer the jam to a heatproof airtight container and let cool completely.

☆ **MAKE AHEAD**
The jam will keep in a jar or airtight container in the refrigerator for up to 1 week.

NUTRITION INFORMATION (1 TABLESPOON):
Calories: 13 | Added sugar: ¼ teaspoon or 1g | Carbohydrates: 3g | Sodium: <1mg | Saturated fat: 0% of calories or 0g | Fiber: <1g | Protein: 1g

MAPLE-VANILLA WHIPPED CREAM

OURS: 0 TEASPOONS*
THEIRS: ¼ TEASPOON

A touch of maple syrup and vanilla boost the flavor in this whipped cream with just a negligible amount of added sugar. It's delicious atop Caramelized Pumpkin Pie (page 148), Blueberry Pie (page 144), and Pumpkin Spice Hot Chocolate (page 174). Remember that although this recipe is made with less sugar, it's still high in saturated fat because of the cream. Use sparingly and balance the remainder of your meals throughout the day to account for this special treat.

Place the cream in the chilled bowl of a stand mixer fitted with a whisk attachment, and beat on medium speed until soft peaks form, about 3 minutes. Add the maple syrup and vanilla and beat on medium-high speed until medium-to-stiff peaks form, about 30 seconds more. Serve immediately.

NUTRITION INFORMATION (2 TABLESPOONS):
Calories: 53 | Added sugar: 0 teaspoons or 0g | Carbohydrates: 1g | Sodium: 4mg | Saturated fat: 58% of calories or 3g | Fiber: 0g | Protein: <1g

*Negligible

Ingredients

1 cup heavy (whipping) cream
1½ teaspoons maple syrup
½ teaspoon pure vanilla extract

MAKES 2 CUPS

SALTED MAPLE-DATE CARAMEL SAUCE

OURS: 1¾ TEASPOONS
THEIRS: 4¾ TO 6 TEASPOONS

Ingredients

8 ounces Medjool dates, pitted (about 10 dates)
1½ cups hot water
1 cup whole milk or almond milk
½ cup maple syrup
½ teaspoon pure vanilla extract
Dash of flaky sea salt

MAKES ABOUT 1¼ CUPS

Naturally sweet dates add caramel flavor with two thirds less sugar than packaged salted caramel sauce. This recipe is great swirled into ice cream (see page 164), with Molten Chocolate Cakes (page 157), or as a topping for waffles and pancakes.

1 Place the dates in a medium bowl and cover with the hot water. Soak until very soft, 10 to 15 minutes, then drain.

2 Transfer the dates to a small saucepan, add the milk and maple syrup, and bring to a low boil, stirring constantly. Reduce the heat to low and simmer and cook until the dates start to break apart, about 5 minutes, watching closely and stirring occasionally so the milk doesn't burn. Remove from the heat and add the vanilla. Let the mixture cool briefly.

3 Place in a food processor or blender and puree, scraping the side of the bowl a few times, until very smooth and no chunks of date remain, about 1 minute. Add the salt, then blend again. Serve warm or cool.

☆ **MAKE AHEAD**
The sauce will keep in a jar or airtight container in the refrigerator for several weeks.

NUTRITION INFORMATION (2 TABLESPOONS):
Calories: 85 | Added sugar: 1¾ teaspoons or 7g | Carbohydrates: 21g | Sodium: 20mg | Saturated fat: 3% of calories or <1g | Fiber: 1g | Protein: 1g

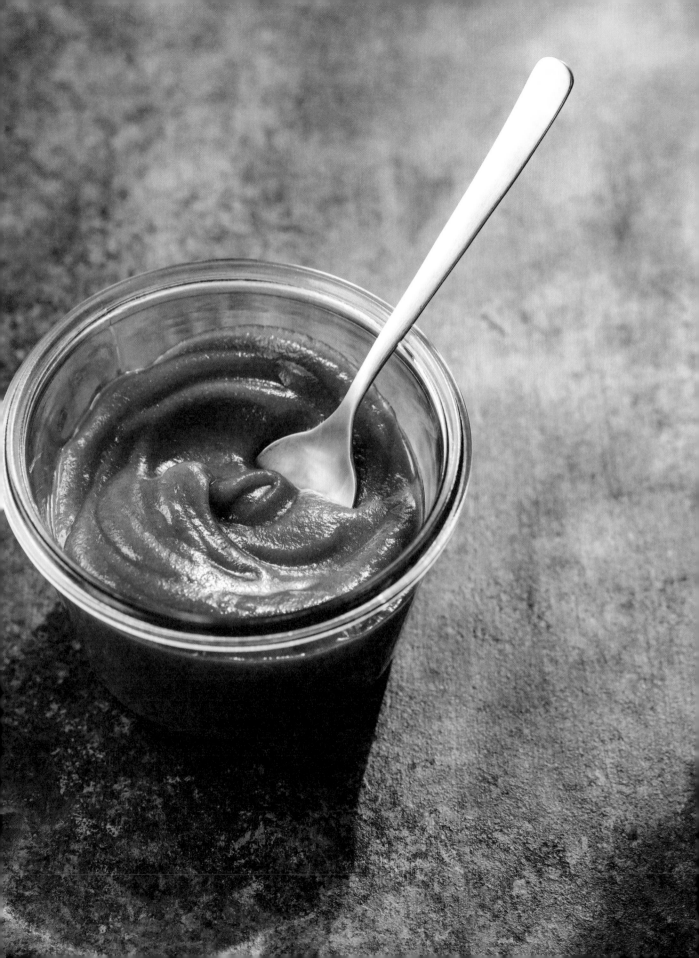

OVERNIGHT PIZZA DOUGH

OURS = 0 TEASPOONS
THEIRS = ½ TO 1 TEASPOON

Ingredients

½ teaspoon active dry
    yeast (see Quick Tip)
½ cup warm water
    (105°F to 115°F)
1 teaspoon extra-virgin
    olive oil
¼ cup room-temperature
    water
2 cups all-purpose flour,
    plus extra as needed
½ teaspoon salt
Nonstick cooking spray

MAKES ABOUT 1 POUND

⚡ QUICK TIP

To make the pizza on the
same day that you make
the dough, increase the
amount of active dry
yeast to 1 teaspoon.
After kneading the
dough, place in an oiled
bowl, cover with plastic
wrap, and let rise in a
warm spot until doubled
in size, about 1 hour.
At this point, you can
continue with Step 4
or, if you're not ready to
bake yet, refrigerate the
dough for up to 6 hours
and then continue with
Step 4.

Letting pizza dough rise overnight in the refrigerator means less
babysitting than when you make it the same day, plus the dough
develops extra flavor during this slow fermentation. This recipe
gives you two options for kneading the dough, depending on what
equipment and how much time you have (the food processor
is easiest and fastest). This makes enough dough for our BBQ
Chicken Pizza (page 124) or Spinach-Ricotta Calzones (page 127).

1 Mix together the yeast and
    warm water in a small bowl.
Cover with a clean dish towel
and let sit until thick and cloudy,
20 minutes. Stir in the olive oil
and room-temperature water.

2 Place the flour and salt in a food
    processor and pulse to combine.
Add the yeast mixture and pulse
until it forms into a ball. Process
until smooth and elastic, another
30 seconds. Transfer to a floured
surface and knead a few times
until smooth.

3 Lightly coat a large bowl or large
    plastic container with cooking
spray. Form the dough into a ball
and place in the bowl. Cover with
plastic wrap and refrigerate for 16
to 24 hours.

4 At least 35 minutes before
    assembling the pizza, remove
the dough from the refrigerator,
punch it down, and re-form it into
a ball. Proceed as directed in the
pizza or calzone recipe.

VARIATION:

To mix and knead by hand: Whisk
together the flour and salt in
a large bowl. Stir in the yeast
mixture and mix until it forms a
dough. Gather up the dough and
transfer to a floured surface, then
knead until very stretchy and
smooth, about 10 minutes. If the
dough gets sticky, add more flour,
1 tablespoon at a time. Continue
with Step 3.

NUTRITION INFORMATION (ABOUT 3 OUNCES UNCOOKED):
Calories: 191 | Added sugar: 0 teaspoons or 0g | Carbohydrates: 38g | Sodium: 235mg |
Saturated fat: 1% of calories or <1g | Fiber: 2g | Protein: 5g

PASTRY DOUGH

This no-added-sugar pie crust gets its flaky texture from apple cider vinegar. It's great to have on hand in the fridge or freezer.

1 Combine ¼ cup water with the vinegar in a small measuring cup. Place the flour and salt in a food processor and pulse to mix. Add the butter and pulse again until the mixture is the texture of coarse cornmeal, about 30 seconds. Add ice to the water-vinegar mixture to chill, then drizzle 3 tablespoons onto the flour mixture. Pulse until a dough forms, about 30 seconds more. Add more of the water-vinegar mixture, a teaspoon at a time, if you need it.

2 Transfer the dough to a clean work surface. Gather the dough into a ball, then divide it in half and flatten each half into a thick disk.

Wrap tightly in plastic wrap and chill in the refrigerator for at least 30 minutes before using.

3 To roll out a crust, dust a rolling pin and work surface with flour. Unwrap a disk of dough and set it on the surface. Roll it into a circle about 12 inches in diameter and ⅛ inch thick. Carefully transfer it to an 8- or 9-inch pie plate and, using your fingers, press the dough into the pie plate and up the side, allowing the dough to hang off the edge. Use scissors to trim excess dough, leaving a ½ inch overhang. Tuck the dough overhang under itself and use the back of a fork to crimp the edge.

Ingredients

1 teaspoon apple cider vinegar

2 cups all-purpose flour, plus extra for rolling out the dough

1 teaspoon salt

1 cup (2 sticks) cold unsalted butter, cut into pieces

1 or 2 ice cubes

MAKES 2 CRUSTS

⚡ QUICK TIP
If you wish to top the pie with dough cutouts, reroll the scraps and cut them into shapes with cookie cutters.

☆ MAKE AHEAD
The dough will keep, tightly wrapped in plastic wrap, in the refrigerator for up to 3 days or in the freezer for up to 1 month.

NUTRITION INFORMATION (⅛ CRUST):
Calories: 159 | Added sugar: 0 teaspoons or 0g | Carbohydrates: 12g | Sodium: 147mg | Saturated fat: 41% of calories or 7g | Fiber: 0g | Protein: 2g

ABOUT BLIND BAKING

When a crust will be filled with a wet or unbaked filling, it must first be blind baked—that is, baked unfilled—to keep it from getting soggy. To blind bake a crust, line it with a round of parchment paper (cut to the diameter of the pan), then fill it with pie weights or dry rice. Bake at 350°F for 15 minutes, then lift out the parchment and weights and prick the bottom of the crust all over with a fork. Return the crust to the oven and continue baking until it is golden brown, about 5 minutes longer. Proceed with the recipe as directed.

CONVERSION TABLES

Please note that all conversions are approximate but close enough to be useful when converting from one system to another.

OVEN TEMPERATURES

FAHRENHEIT	GAS MARK	CELSIUS
250	½	120
275	1	140
300	2	150
325	3	160
350	4	180
375	5	190
400	6	200
425	7	220
450	8	230
475	9	240
500	10	260

Note: Reduce the temperature by 20°C (68°F) for fan-assisted ovens.

APPROXIMATE EQUIVALENTS

1 stick butter = 8 tbs = 4 oz = ½ cup = 115 g

1 cup all-purpose presifted flour = 4.7 oz

1 cup granulated sugar = 8 oz = 220 g

1 cup (firmly packed) brown sugar = 6 oz = 220 to 230 g

1 cup confectioners' sugar = 4½ oz = 115 g

1 cup honey or syrup = 12 oz

1 cup grated cheese = 4 oz

1 cup dried beans = 6 oz

1 large egg = about 2 oz or about 3 tbs

1 egg yolk = about 1 tbs

1 egg white = about 2 tbs

LIQUID CONVERSIONS

US	IMPERIAL	METRIC
2 tbs.	1 fl oz	30 ml
3 tbs.	1½ fl oz	45 ml
¼ cup	2 fl oz	60 ml
⅓ cup	2½ fl oz	75 ml
⅓ cup + 1 tbs	3 fl oz	90 ml
⅓ cup + 2 tbs	3½ fl oz	100 ml
½ cup	4 fl oz	125 ml
⅔ cup	5 fl oz	150 ml
¾ cup	6 fl oz	175 ml
¾ cup + 2 tbs	7 fl oz	200 ml
1 cup	8 fl oz	250 ml
1 cup + 2 tbs	9 fl oz	275 ml
1¼ cups	10 fl oz	300 ml
1⅓ cups	11 fl oz	325 ml
1½ cups	12 fl oz	350 ml
1⅔ cups	13 fl oz	375 ml
1¾ cups	14 fl oz	400 ml
1¾ cups + 2 tbs.	15 fl oz	450 ml
2 cups (1 pint)	16 fl oz	500 ml
2½ cups	20 fl oz (1 pint)	600 ml
3¾ cups	1½ pints	900 ml
4 cups (1 quart)	1¾ pints	1 liter

WEIGHT CONVERSIONS

US/UK	METRIC	US/UK	METRIC
½ oz	15 g	7 oz	200 g
1 oz	30 g	8 oz	250 g
1½ oz	45 g	9 oz	275 g
2 oz	60 g	10 oz	300 g
2½ oz	75 g	11 oz	325 g
3 oz	90 g	12 oz	350 g
3½ oz	100 g	13 oz	375 g
4 oz	125 g	14 oz	400 g
5 oz	150 g	15 oz	450 g
6 oz	175 g	1 lb	500 g

Acknowledgments

It truly takes a team to bring a book to life. We are grateful to the many people who helped along the way.

Danielle Svetcov's dedication to our mission was instrumental in making this book a reality. We couldn't have done it without her, and we are incredibly thankful for her steadfast support.

A heartfelt thank you to Susan Bolotin, Kylie Foxx McDonald, and the entire team at Workman Publishing, who have been a dream team to work with. Kylie supported this idea from the start and led the charge tirelessly, with Becky Terhune, Ann Taylor Pittman, Sarah Curley, Donna Ingram, Kate Karol, and Barbara Peragine to make this book an invaluable resource for busy families. Rebecca Carlisle, Moira Kerrigan, Chloe Puton, and Erin Kibby, together with the amazing Kate Bittman, were instrumental in getting the word out for us, and we are grateful for their passionate support.

As any experienced cook knows, cutting out sugar and keeping the flavor in our favorite foods is a feat. An amazing team of talented chefs rose to the challenge to refine and test the recipes in this book. Tara Duggan, Isabelle English, and Sandra Wu spent a year testing recipes and were top-notch teammates in the kitchen. Our cravings are satisfied thanks to their hard work. Laura Vollmer helped us ensure that all of the recipes met our nutritional standards. And to all of our family members, friends, and colleagues who provided feedback and tasted the recipes in this book, we are thankful for all that you did to help.

Our amazing creative team of Erin Scott, Lillian Kang, Ashley Lima, Nicola Parisi, Nick Wolf, Veronica Laramie, and Shawn Burke helped us create the beautiful pictures in these pages. Their talent makes it easy to show that you don't have to give up the foods you love to reduce sugar.

Because of our families, we get to share this book with you. To them we owe the biggest thanks. Our children were our inspiration. James, Catherine, Kasmira, and Iyla cooked recipes, shared feedback, and were enthusiastic taste testers. We are so thankful for their love of food and cooking. Our husbands, Anthony and Sam, supported us every step of the way. Without them this book would simply be an idea. And to our parents, a lifetime of gratitude. Your commitment to bringing family around the table to share a good meal inspired us to do the same.

Like they did for us, we hope these recipes will help you nourish your family, bring friends and family together to make wonderful memories, and enjoy all of the foods you love in a healthier way.

—Jennifer and Anisha

ENDNOTES

and leads to better performance at school: T. Burrows, et al., "Is There an Association Between Dietary Intake and Academic Achievement: A Systematic Review." *Journal of Human Nutrition and Dietetics: The Official Journal of the British Dietetic Association* 30, no. 2 (2017): 117–140, https://doi.org/10.1111/jhn12407.

an ingredient that is undermining the health of our families: added sugar: M. B. Vos et al., "Added Sugars and Cardiovascular Disease Risk in Children: A Scientific Statement from the American Heart Association," *Circulation* 135, no. 19 (2017): e1017–e1034, https://doi.org/10.1161/CIR.0000000000000439.

Half of it comes from sugary drinks. The other half is in the foods they eat: M. B. Vos et al., "Added Sugars and Cardiovascular Disease Risk in Children: A Scientific Statement from the American Heart Association," *Circulation* 135, no. 19 (2017): e1017–e1034, https://doi.org/10.1161/CIR.0000000000000439.

Scientific studies increasingly point to the health harms of sugar: M. B. Vos et al., "Added Sugars and Cardiovascular Disease Risk in Children: A Scientific Statement from the American Heart Association," *Circulation* 135, no. 19 (2017): e1017–e1034, https://doi.org/10.1161/CIR.0000000000000439.

including obesity, type 2 diabetes, high blood pressure, and abnormal cholesterol levels: M. B. Vos et al., "Added Sugars and Cardiovascular Disease Risk in Children: A Scientific Statement from the American Heart Association," *Circulation* 135, no. 19 (2017): e1017–e1034, https://doi.org/10.1161/CIR.0000000000000439.

V. S. Malik, "Sugar Sweetened Beverages and Cardiometabolic Health," *Current Opinion in Cardiology* 32, no. 5 (2017): 572–579, https://doi.org/10.1097/hco.0000000000000439.

Added sugar can also cause fatty liver disease, which can lead to liver failure: M. B. Vos et al., "Added Sugars and Cardiovascular Disease Risk in Children: A Scientific Statement from the American Heart Association," *Circulation* 135, no. 19 (2017): e1017–e1034, https://doi.org/10.1161/CIR.0000000000000439.

V. S. Malik, "Sugar Sweetened Beverages and Cardiometabolic Health," *Current Opinion in Cardiology* 32, no. 5 (2017): 572–579, https://doi.org/10.1097/hco.0000000000000439.

diseases that are the leading causes of death in the United States: L. J. Collin et al., "Association of Sugary Beverage Consumption with Mortality Risk in US Adults: A Secondary Analysis of Data from the REGARDS Study," *JAMA Network Open* 2, no. 5 (May 17, 2019): e193121, https://doi.org/10.1001/jamanetworkopen.2019.3121.

obesity rates in this age group increasing at an alarming rate: A. C. Skinner et al., "Prevalence of Obesity and Severe Obesity in US Children, 1999–2016," *Pediatrics* 141, no. 3 (2018): e20173459, https://doi.org/10.1542/peds.2017-3459.

the leading chronic health condition among children: P. Moynihan, "Sugars and Dental Caries: Evidence for Setting a Recommended Threshold for Intake," *Advances in Nutrition* 7, no. 1 (2016):149–156, https://doi.org/10.3945/an.115.009365.

three times the recommended daily limit of added sugar: M. B. Vos et al., "Added Sugars and Cardiovascular Disease Risk in Children: A Scientific Statement from the American Heart Association," *Circulation* 135, no. 19 (2017): e1017–e1034, https://doi.org/10.1161/CIR.0000000000000439.

R. K. Johnson, et al., "Dietary Sugars Intake and Cardiovascular Health: A Scientific Statement from the American Heart Association," *Circulation* 120, no. 11 (2009):1011–20, https://doi.org/10.1161/CIRCULATIONAHA.109.192627.

will influence behavior when they're older: C. A. Forestell, "Flavor Perception and Preference Development in Human Infants," *Annals of Nutrition and Metabolism* 3, supplement 3 (2017):17–25, https://doi.org/10.1159/000478759.

may be able to reverse these conditions by eating a low-sugar diet: J. B. Schwimmer et al., "Effect of a Low Free Sugar Diet vs Usual Diet on Nonalcoholic Fatty Liver Disease in Adolescent Boys: A Randomized Clinical Trial," *JAMA* 321, no. 3 (2019): 256–265, https://doi.org/10.1001/jama.2018.20579.

R. H. Lustig et al., "Isocaloric Fructose Restriction and Metabolic Improvement in Children with Obesity and Metabolic Syndrome," *Obesity* 24, no. 2 (2016): 453–460, https://doi.org/10.1002/oby.21371.

Most added sugars are consumed at home: R. B. Ervin et al., "Consumption of Added Sugar Among U.S. Children and Adolescents, 2005–2008," *National Center for Health Statistics Data Brief* 87 (March 2012): 1–8, https://www.cdc.gov/nchs/data/databriefs/db87.pdf.

does not consider fruit juice added sugar: M. B. Vos et al., "Added Sugars and Cardiovascular Disease Risk in Children: A Scientific Statement from the American Heart Association," *Circulation* 135, no.19 (2017): e1017–e1034, https://doi.org/10.1161/CIR.0000000000000439.

counts both fruit juice and fruit juice concentrates as added sugar: World Health Organization, *Guideline: Sugars intake for adults and children* (2015), accessed May 27, 2019, https://who.int/nutrition/publications/guidelines/sugars_intake/en/.

what happens when you drink a can of soda: Fig. 1 by University of California, "What Does Sugar Actually Do to Your Body?", accessed May 27, 2019, https://youtube.com/watch?v=utXcI3FqzeM.

Soda primarily contains two types of sugar: fructose and glucose. There is some variation in how the body processes different types of sugar. Although high-fructose corn syrup is processed somewhat differently than table sugar, research suggests that excessive consumption of all added sugar is harmful to health.

experienced improvements in waist size, body fat, blood sugar, and blood pressure levels: C. D. Gardner et al., "Effect of Low-Fat vs Low-Carbohydrate Diet on 12-Month Weight Loss in Overweight Adults and the Association with Genotype Pattern or Insulin Secretion: The DIETFITS Randomized Clinical Trial," *JAMA* 319, no. 7 (2018): 667–679, https://doi.org/10.1001/jama.2018.0245.

and use of minimal amounts of sugar, salt, and fats to flavor foods:
Council on School Health, Committee on Nutrition, "Snacks, Sweetened
Beverages, Added Sugars, and Schools." *Pediatrics* 135, no. 3 (2015):
575–583, https://doi.org/10.1542/peds.2014-3902.

**do not have healthier weights, have lower self-esteem, and are at risk for
eating disorders:** Academy of Nutrition and Dietetics, "Helping Kids Maintain
a Healthy Body Weight: A Cheat Sheet for Success, accessed May 27, 2019,
https://eatright.org/health/weight-loss/your-health-and-your-weight/helping-
kids-maintain-a-healthy-body-weight-a-cheat-sheet-for-success.

Sugar goes by more than sixty different names (see page 2): "Hidden in
Plain Sight," SugarScience, University of California, San Francisco, accessed
May 27, 2019, http://sugarscience.ucsf.edu/hidden-in-plain-sight
/#.XOx7b4hKg2w.

proteins, antioxidants, and micronutrients: E. M. Whitaker, "The Sweet
Science of Honey," SugarScience, University of California, San Francisco,
accessed May 27, 2019, http://sugarscience.ucsf.edu/the-sweet-science-
behind-honey.html#.XOxr2ohKg2w.

and is recommended as a remedy for cough: O. Oduwole et al., "Honey for
Acute Cough in Children," *The Cochrane Database of Systematic Reviews* 4
(2018): CD007094, https://doi.org/10.1002/14651858.CD007094.pub5.

essentially the same once fully processed by the body: There is some variation
in how the body processes different types of sugar. Although high-fructose corn
syrup is processed somewhat differently than table sugar, research suggests that
excessive consumption of all added sugar is harmful to health.

count toward your daily sugar limit (see page 10): Due to concerns regarding
botulism, honey should never be given to infants less than 12 months of age.

children are not eating the recommended amount of fruit and vegetables:
S. A. Kim et al., "Vital Signs: Fruit and Vegetable Intake Among Children—
United States, 2003–2010," *Morbidity and Mortality Weekly Report,* 63, no.
31 (2014): 671–676, https://ncbi.nlm.nih.gov/pubmed/25102415.

and that children limit their daily fruit juice consumption: M. B. Heyman
and S. A. Abrams, Section on Gastroenterology, Hepatology, and Nutrition,
Committee on Nutrition. "Fruit Juice in Infants, Children, and Adolescents:
Current Recommendations," *Pediatrics* 139, no. 6 (2017): e20170967,
https://doi.org/10.1542/peds.2017-0967.

and their health harms cannot be excluded:

M. Pearlman, J. Obert, and L. Casey, "The Association Between Artificial
Sweeteners and Obesity," *Current Gastroenterology Reports* 19, no. 12 (2017):
64, https://doi.org/10.1007/s11894-017-0602-9.

S. Duran Aguero et al., "Noncaloric Sweeteners in Children: A Controversial
Theme," *BioMed Research International* 2018: 4806534, https://doi.org
/10.1155/2018/4806534.

play a role in obesity and other health problems: F. J. Ruiz-Ojeda et al.,
"Effects of Sweeteners on the Gut Microbiota: A Review of Experimental
Studies and Clinical Trials," *Advances in Nutrition* 10, supplement 1 (2019):
S31–S48, https://doi.org/10.1093/advances/nmy037.

has not been fully evaluated by the Food and Drug Administration:
"Has Stevia Been Approved by FDA to Be Used as a Sweetener?", U.S.
Food & Drug Administration, accessed May 27, 2019, https://www.fda.gov
/about-fda/fda-basics/has-stevia-been-approved-fda-be-used-sweetener.

(ADI) levels for more long-standing sugar substitutes : For saccharin, for
example, the ADI level is 2.4 (10-ounce) cans of diet soda for a 150-pound
adult and 0.8 of a 12-ounce can for a 50-pound child.

**Half of added sugar intake comes from beverages. Another 20 percent comes
from hidden sugar like that in condiments, dressings, and sauces:** M. B. Vos
et al., "Added Sugars and Cardiovascular Disease Risk in Children: A Scientific
Statement from the American Heart Association," *Circulation* 135, no. 19
(2017): e1017–e1034, https://doi.org/10.1161/CIR.0000000000000439.

How Much Fruit Juice Is Okay?: M. B. Heyman and S. A. Abrams,
Section on Gastroenterology, Hepatology, and Nutrition, Committee
on Nutrition. "Fruit Juice in Infants, Children, and Adolescents: Current
Recommendations," *Pediatrics* 139, no. 6 (2017): e20170967, https://doi
.org/10.1542/peds.2017-0967.

increase hydration to promote learning: C. J. Edmunds et al., "Dose-Response
Effects of Water Supplementation on Cognitive Performance and Mood
in Children and Adults, *Appetite* 108, (January 1, 2017): 464–470,
https://doi.org/10.1016/j.appet.2016.11.011.

**up to 6 teaspoons for children 2 to 18 years old, 6 teaspoons for women,
and 9 teaspoons for men:**

M. B. Vos et al., "Added Sugars and Cardiovascular Disease Risk in
Children: A Scientific Statement from the American Heart Association,"
Circulation 135, no. 19 (2017): e1017–e1034, https://doi.org/10.1161
/CIR.0000000000000439.

R. K. Johnson, et al., "Dietary Sugars Intake and Cardiovascular Health:
A Scientific Statement from the American Heart Association," *Circulation*
120, no. 11 (2009):1011–20, https://doi.org/10.1161/CIRCULATIONAHA
.109.192627.

**should not consume any food or beverages with added sugar, including
sugar-sweetened drinks:** M. B. Vos et al., "Added Sugars and Cardiovascular
Disease Risk in Children: A Scientific Statement from the American Heart
Association," *Circulation* 135, no. 19 (2017): e1017–e1034, https://doi.org
/10.1161/CIR.0000000000000439.

1,500 mg or less of sodium a day for all Americans for ideal heart health:
"How Much Sodium Should I Eat Per Day?", American Heart Association,
accessed May 27, 2019, https://heart.org/en/healthy-living/healthy-eating
/eat-smart/sodium/how-much-sodium-should-i-eat-per-day.

Federal Dietary Guidelines serve as our upper bound: "Dietary Guidelines
for Americans 2015–2020, Eighth Edition," U.S. Department of Health
and Human Services and U.S. Department of Agriculture, accessed
May 27, 2019, https://health.gov/dietaryguidelines/2015/guidelines
/chapter-1/key-recommendations/.

keep saturated fats to 10 percent of total calories per day: "Dietary Guidelines
for Americans 2015–2020, Eighth Edition," U.S. Department of Health
and Human Services and U.S. Department of Agriculture, accessed
May 27, 2019, https://health.gov/dietaryguidelines/2015/guidelines
/chapter-1/key-recommendations/.

INDEX

pork roast, Chinese, sweet and
    sticky (char siu), 108
potato chips, baked, 62
pulled pork sliders with tangy
    buttermilk apple slaw, 105–6,
    107
sauce, *184, 185*
spice mix, *184,* 185
Beans:
    Boston baked, 97
    green, citrus chicken stir-fry with,
        100
Bean sprouts:
    shrimp pad Thai, 119
    Vietnamese chicken noodle soup,
        101
Bear toast, *30,* 33
Beef:
    and broccoli teriyaki bowls,
        109–10
    Gram's meatballs and spaghetti,
        126
    pineapple teriyaki short ribs,
        111–13, *112*
    sloppy joes, 114
Beverages:
    blueberry-almond smoothie,
        179, 181
    caramel coffee frappé, 170
    horchata, 175
    hot chocolate blocks, *172,* 173
    kids' chocolate frappé, 171
    mango-pineapple smoothie,
        178, 179
    pumpkin spice hot chocolate, 174
    strawberry-cantaloupe agua
        fresca, 176
    strawberry-peach smoothie,
        177, 179
Blind baking crust for pies, 203
Blondies with white chocolate and
    almonds, 135
Blood sugar, 4
Blueberry(ies):
    -almond smoothie, *179,* 181
    bear toast, *30,* 33
    monkey toast, *30, 31*
    -oat muffins, 45–46, *47*
    owl toast, *30, 32*
    pie, 144, *145*
    scones, 39–40, *41*

Boston baked beans, 97
Breads:
    banana, super moist, 52, *53*
    bear toast, *30,* 33
    caramelized pumpkin, 50, *51*
    maple–brown butter corn, *54, 55*
    monkey toast, *30, 31*
    overnight French toast strata with
        raspberry sauce, 37–38
    owl toast, *30, 32*
Breakfast dishes:
    apple-cinnamon instant oatmeal,
        24, 25–26
    banana-chocolate muffins, 48–49
    bear toast, *30,* 33
    blueberry-oat muffins, 45–46, *47*
    blueberry scones, 39–40, *41*
    caramelized pumpkin bread, *50,*
        51
    cherry-oatmeal breakfast cookies,
        20–21
    cinnamon-apple coffee cake,
        42, 43–44
    fruit and nut granola, 22, *23*
    health benefits, 8
    honey-peach breakfast pops,
        18, 19
    maple–brown butter corn bread,
        54, 55
    monkey toast, *30, 31*
    overnight French toast strata with
        raspberry sauce, 37–38
    owl toast, *30, 32*
    pumpkin spice waffles with maple
        yogurt, *34,* 35–36
    strawberry toaster pastries,
        27–28, *29*
    super moist banana bread, 52, *53*
Broccoli and beef teriyaki bowls,
    109–10
Brownies, double chocolate,
    136, 137
Brown sugar:
    buying, 13
    grams of sugar in, 11
Brussels sprouts:
    fall harvest Mason jar salad with
        creamy poppy seed dressing,
        82–84, *83*
Burgers, pineapple teriyaki salmon,
    with sriracha mayo, 120

C

Cabbage:
    BBQ pulled pork sliders with
        tangy buttermilk apple slaw,
        105–6, *107*
    Chinese chicken salad with
        Mandarin vinaigrette, 85
    shrimp pad Thai, 119
Cakes:
    chocolate and peanut butter
        snack, *150,* 151–52
    cinnamon-apple coffee, *42,*
        43–44
    double chocolate layer, with
        whipped chocolate frosting,
        158–60, *159*
    red velvet cupcakes with cream
        cheese frosting, 153–54, *155*
    salted maple-date caramel molten
        chocolate, *156,* 157
Calzones, spinach-ricotta, 127
Cantaloupe-strawberry agua fresca,
    176
Caramel:
    coffee frappé, 170
    corn, maple, *64,* 65
    salted, and chocolate, no-churn
        banana ice cream with, 164, *165*
    salted, chocolate cheesecake bars,
        138–39
    salted maple-date, molten
        chocolate cakes, *156,* 157
    sauce, salted maple-date, 200, *201*
Caramelized pumpkin bread, *50,* 51
Caramelized pumpkin pie, 148, *149*
Carrots:
    alphabet soup, 79
    BBQ pulled pork sliders with
        tangy buttermilk apple slaw,
        105–6, *107*
    cherry-oatmeal breakfast cookies,
        20–21
    Chinese BBQ pork fried rice, 78
    cold sesame noodles with tofu and
        vegetables, 77
    creamy tomato soup, *80, 81*
    pineapple teriyaki short ribs,
        111–13, *112*
    shrimp pad Thai, 119

Crispy rice treats, salted nut butter, 140, *141*

Cucumbers:
BBQ chicken chopped salad with creamy ranch dressing, *86*, 87
cold sesame noodles with tofu and vegetables, 77
poke bowls, 116–18, *117*

Cupcakes, red velvet, with cream cheese frosting, 153–54, *155*

D

Date(s):
about, 13
apple-cinnamon instant oatmeal, *24*, 25–26
blondies with white chocolate and almonds, 135
blueberry-oat muffins, 45–46, *47*
caramel coffee frappé, 170
chewy chocolate chip cookies, *130*, 131–32
chocolate and peanut butter snack cake, *150*, 151–52
horchata, 175
ketchup, 190
kids' chocolate frappé, 171
-maple salted caramel molten chocolate cakes, *156*, 157
-maple salted caramel sauce, 200, *201*
no-bake peanut butter energy bars, *58*, 59
peanut butter cookies, 133–34
salted caramel chocolate cheesecake bars, 138–39
super moist banana bread, 52, *53*
sweet and spicy chile sauce, 94
sweet soy-garlic sauce, 95

Desserts:
added sugars in, 6
apple crisp, *146*, 147
blondies with white chocolate and almonds, 135
blueberry pie, 144, *145*
caramelized pumpkin pie, 148, *149*
chai-spiced rice pudding, 161
chewy chocolate chip cookies, *130*, 131–32

chocolate and peanut butter snack cake, *150*, 151–52
chocolate pudding with maple-vanilla whipped cream, *162*, 163
double chocolate brownies, *136*, 137
double chocolate layer cake with whipped chocolate frosting, 158–60, *159*
no-churn banana ice cream with chocolate and salted caramel, 164, *165*
peanut butter cookies, 133–34
pecan pie bars, *142*, 143
red velvet cupcakes with cream cheese frosting, 153–54, *155*
salted caramel chocolate cheesecake bars, 138–39
salted maple-date caramel molten chocolate cakes, *156*, 157
salted nut butter crispy rice treats, 140, *141*
strawberry cream pops, *166*, 167

Dinners:
BBQ chicken pizza, 124, *125*
BBQ chicken with grilled corn salad, 96–97
BBQ pulled pork sliders with tangy buttermilk apple slaw, 105–6, *107*
beef and broccoli teriyaki bowls, 109–10
Boston baked beans, 97
Chinese chicken lettuce cups, 98, *99*
citrus chicken stir-fry with green beans, 100
Gram's meatballs and spaghetti, 126
miso-glazed salmon, 115
oven-baked Korean chicken wings, *92*, 93
pineapple teriyaki salmon burgers with sriracha mayo, 120
pineapple teriyaki short ribs, 111–13, *112*
poke bowls, 116–18, *117*
rainbow chard lasagna, 121–23, *122*
shrimp pad Thai, 119
sloppy joes, 114

spinach-ricotta calzones, 127
stuffed chicken Parmesan strips with 5-minute marinara dipping sauce, *102*, 103–4
sweet and sticky Chinese BBQ pork roast (char siu), 108

Double chocolate brownies, *136*, 137

Double chocolate layer cake with whipped chocolate frosting, 158–60, *159*

Dressings:
creamy poppy seed, 194
creamy ranch, 192
mandarin vinaigrette, 193
roasted strawberry balsamic vinaigrette, 195

E

Egg(s):
Chinese BBQ pork fried rice, 78
shrimp pad Thai, 119
yolks, for recipes, 13

Energy bars, no-bake peanut butter, *58*, 59

F

Fall harvest Mason jar salad with creamy poppy seed dressing, 82–84, *83*

Farro:
fall harvest Mason jar salad with creamy poppy seed dressing, 82–84, *83*

Fats, dietary, 11

Fiber:
benefits of, 4
in fruits and vegetables, 8

Fish:
miso-glazed salmon, 115
pineapple teriyaki salmon burgers with sriracha mayo, 120
poke bowls, 116–18, *117*
salmon yaki onigiri (grilled rice balls), 74–76, *75*

5-minute marinara dipping sauce, *102*, 104